Dear Couch,
We're Through!

SHIRES ● PRESS

4869 Main Street | Manchester Center, VT 05255 | www.northshire.com

Dear Couch, We're Through!

How to get started, stay motivated, & have fun with your exercise.

©2018 by J E N N   B E N S O N

ISBN: 978-0-9964842-3-7

www.jennbenson.com

Author's Note: The information in this book is comprised of opinion, personal experience, research, and personal suggestions. Mention of companies, websites, organizations, and authorities do not endorse the author. Names, characters, places, and incidents are a product of the author's imagination or experience. Locales and public names are sometimes used for atmospheric purposes. Any resemblance to actual people, living or dead, or to businesses, companies, events, institutions, or locales is completely coincidental.

Special thanks to Lauren Hull for cover and author photo (www. laurenhullphotography.com), Debbi Wraga for her awesome book design, my editing team Samantha Williams (www.samanthaedenwilliams.com) and Aubrey Restifo, Michelle Lanne and Jessica Pfitzner for their literary genius and expertise, and lastly, my wonderful clients for inspiring me to do this and always finding new ways to keep moving forward!

NORTHSHIRE BOOKSTORE
Building Community, One Book at a Time

A family-owned, independent bookstore in Manchester Ctr., VT, since 1976 and Saratoga Springs, NY since 2013.
We are committed to excellence in bookselling. The Northshire Bookstore's mission is to serve as a resource for information, ideas, and entertainment while honoring the needs of customers, staff, and community.

Printed in the United States of America

Dear Couch, We're Through!

How to get started, stay motivated,
& have fun with your exercise.

JENN BENSON

SHIRES **PRESS**

Dear Couch,

We're Through! I have wasted enough of my life sitting around with you. It is clear to see that you and I are going nowhere. It's time for me to get a move on. Gotta get going!

Me

"No matter how slow you go,
you are still lapping everybody on the couch."

Contents

Contents (CONTINUED)

PART 3: HAVING FUN
Enjoying Exercise, Your New Soul Mate

Contents (CONTINUED)

Introduction

The Breakup

Introduction
_____

The Breakup

It is proven that daily exercise improves your mood, boosts energy, controls weight, combats disease, relieves stress, improves learning, builds self-esteem, eases back pain, fights dementia, prevents muscle loss, improves oxygen supply, detoxifies the body, improves sex life, increases endurance, improves joint function, lowers blood pressure, lowers diabetes risk, improves posture, improves concentration, enhances cardiovascular function, increases metabolic rate, aids in digestion, eases muscular tension, regulates hormones, reduces pain and irritability, reduces inflammation—AND enhances our lives in too many other ways to list! I know what you may be thinking. Blah, blah, blah because most of us already know all of these benefits. Why is it, then, that we find it so difficult to make exercise a priority in our lives? What is so darn hard about getting up and moving around?

We all know those bizarre people who get their daily dose of exercise no matter what. They always seem so enthusiastic about it, too! You have to wonder: what makes them so special? What in the world is their motivation? Have they always loved to pump iron at the gym? Have they always enjoyed getting up at the crack of dawn to run a gazillion miles? Chances are these avid exercise freaks had to, at some point in their lives, silence their inner couch potato and ignore *"Couch"* (as I will refer to it in this book) and its sneaky seduction. It all starts with a mission.

We all have Couch—the office chair, the driver's seat, that dorm study hall, that favorite "lounge around" piece of furniture into which we sink and feel as if we could be fine if we never got up again. *"Couch"* is quite simply that place where you often plant your butt. The sad fact is, most of what we do on any given day involves a boat load of sitting. In the book, *Get Up!* written by James Levine, MD, he explains that for every hour we sit, we lose two hours of life. Yuck! Now that you know this, doesn't it make you want to get up and move around? The truth is, "sitting disease" is real—and it's killing people. Our relationship with Couch is not healthy for anyone involved.

I agree there will be legitimate reasons for not exercising from time to time, but I am willing to bet that ninety percent of those reasons are lousy, waste-of-our-breath excuses. These excuses will end up limiting us in the future and decreasing the fun factor (which is no fun, by the way!). Lack of exercise consistency and a lifetime of "yo-yo" fitness can happen to all of us. Just be aware that Couch will always be trying to brainwash you. Think of the times we have said, *"My job requires sitting all day, and there is nothing I can do about it,"* or, *"I just want to get home and collapse on the couch."* Yes, I agree these may be true statements. But these are not insurmountable obstacles, right? We all have to make a conscious effort to commit to exercise, even me. Newsflash: We are all human, and this is real life. I am here to tell you it will be challenging at first. it will take some effort, and you may even buckle a few times. Some of you may have a louder, more insistent couch potato person inside your head. But don't worry-there's an app for that!

If you are part of the I-know-exercise-is-good-for-me, but-I-just-can't-bring-myself-to-do-it" club, you are not alone. You may hate those exercising freaks of nature now, but realize that after you read this, you may become one of them yourself. Exercise does not have to be an activity that makes you cringe. It can be fun and very fulfilling. It's time to say good-bye to Couch and start planning for some serious couch pillows to be thrown at you. This breakup may be messy, but it will be totally worth it! A true, active, healthy lifestyle is far more rewarding than the couch potato life can ever hope to be.

In these pages, I will introduce you to my favorite tools and resources that will help you end your needy relationship with Couch. My intention is for you to be happy with who you are, what you look like, and how you feel. Along the way, I will share my own personal experiences in addition to what I have learned over the years from mentors and my own clients. My hope is that you start to feel good and feel confident that YOU CAN stick to an exercise plan that you actually enjoy. So lace up your sneakers, and let's start this adventure by walking out your front door!

We are all human, and this is real life.

I am here to tell you it will be challenging at first. It will take some effort, and you may even buckle a few times.

But don't worry–there's an app for that!

PART 1

Getting Started

Ending Your Relationship with Couch

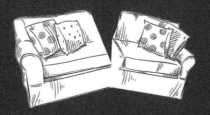

CHAPTER 1

The Final K.I.S.S.

*"You don't have to be great to start,
but you do have to start to be great."*
—*Zig Ziglar*

Kissing Couch good-bye can be tough. That's why it needs to be a small, simple peck on the armrest. When we "Keep It Simple, Sexy," or K.I.S.S. Couch good-bye, we allow ourselves to put small, manageable changes in play that are sure to give Couch the boot for good. One thing I discovered when I started my personal training business was that starting with small changes worked best for most clients, regardless of age, weight, marital status, career, and so forth. The go-big-or-go-home approach doesn't work. We have enough big problems, big deadlines, big shoes to fill, and big aspirations in our lives. Do we really need *"go big"* all of the time (well, maybe if it's a paycheck!)? It's certainly not *"go-big-or-do-nothing"* when it comes to the exercise world! When things seem too big and overwhelming, procrastination rears its despicable head. Small and consistent changes can prevent you from getting bogged down by the pressure of becoming healthy and fit. As Jeff Olson writes in his bestseller *The Slight Edge*, "Do one thing, and you shall have the power." After all, how do you eat an elephant? That's right-one bite at a time.

Getting started with any new endeavor is the hardest part. I mean, things are hard before they get easy, right? Whether you are starting your fitness journey over again or you have never exercised a day in your life, you will probably find that thinking about exercise is easy, talking about it is tough, and taking the first call-to-action step is the hardest part. If you realize this fact, breaking up with Couch will be a whole lot easier. Movement and *"exercise"* is a lifestyle—not a label. Stop labeling it and just start moving more. You may be asking, *"OK, how do I get started?"* Read on, my friend. I will give you some tools to help you skip down the small, merry path to exercise heaven.

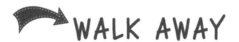WALK AWAY

It takes guts to walk away from Couch. When you start, don't turn around. Just keep going—keep walking. This is a very simple activity that most of us overlook. When you have no idea what to do for exercise or how to start exercising, **JUST WALK**. I have clients who reach their weight loss goals by changing one thing and one thing only: they increase how much they walk. By just getting up and completing this functional daily exercise, you can begin to see amazing results. According to the Surgeon General, we should be walking up to 10,000 steps a day to maintain our weight. Just how far is 10,000 steps, you may ask? Well, since 2000-2500 steps equal one mile (depending, of course, on the length of your stride), 10,000 steps works out to be about four to five miles worth of walking each day. Now, this does not mean you have to go out and walk four miles in one fell swoop. Daily activities, such as walking from the parking lot to the grocery store or walking to the mailbox from your doorstep, all add up.

Walking is a very functional part of living. It does not require any equipment; you can do it anywhere; it's free, and most importantly, it is a daily part of life for most people. Benefits of a brisk walk include: improving your mood, maintaining a healthy weight, preventing high blood pressure and type 2 diabetes, improving balance and coordination, strengthening your heart, preventing dementia and osteoporosis, toning your legs and arms, and boosting your energy, to name a few. You have the power in your own stride!

Don't overlook the importance of walking simply because you do it every day. Remember when you were a baby and everyone came to your house to bake you a cake when you took your first steps? It was such a big deal then. You can even get your friends to bake you a cake again (sugar and gluten-free, of course!). Whether you want to lose weight, get cardio conditioning, increase your longevity, or better your overall health, walking will do the trick. Try apps like **MapMyWalk** and **Pedometer++** to get you started.

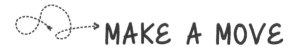

MAKE A MOVE

Remember that annoying kid in class who was always tapping their pencil on their desk or moving around in their seat? That was me, by the way, and my kids have the same gene! *"Just sit still,"* everyone screams. But isn't it better to move *more?*

Dr. James Levine, a researcher at the Mayo Clinic, would say *"yes."* His research on **N.E.A.T.** (Non-Exercise Activity Thermogenesis) basically accounts for all the energy you exert on a daily basis that burns calories outside of eating, sleeping, and deliberate exercise (a.k.a. going to the gym). In other words, the more you move, the more calories you burn. It would make sense then that fidgety people burn more calories. Well, if you ask me, this sounds easy. It's a simple, painless way to burn calories without even stepping foot in the gym. As Nike rightfully puts it in their slogan, we need to *"Just do it."* I would like to change it, however, to *"Just do something."* That tag line probably doesn't fit as well on sweatpants or carry the same flash, but we should try it. Explore some new ways to increase your daily movement, and check them off the list as you go:

☐ Walk to the mailbox to get your mail—don't drive the car up!

☐ March in place during commercials.

☐ Walk, and listen to a book on tape instead of sitting to read it.

☐ Schedule walking meetings or conference calls.

☐ Play fetch with your dog (or crazy cat).

☐ Use a stability ball as your desk chair—super fun and funny!

☐ Take the stairs—no matter what.

☐ Coffee and walk-outings with friends—walk as you sip.

☐ Plan active dates instead of dinner and a movie (hiking, a walk around the neighborhood, or ice skating).

☐ Tour a winery instead of just buying the wine.

☐ Play active games with the kiddos—Wii bowling, anyone?

☐ Get rid of the chairs for your next house party.

☐ Stand while folding laundry.

☐ Go get your food instead of getting delivery.

☐ Squat over your chair for 20 seconds before you sit down.

☐ Drink lots of water—lots of bathroom trips add up.

☐ Stand up every time your phone rings or makes a sound.

☐ Try the app **Move** (you can set reminders and certain times to get you to move) or the app **Stand Up!** (reminds us to do just what it says).

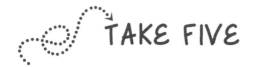

TAKE FIVE

The common misconception when starting an exercise program is that we need to put in hours and miserable hours at the gym. For some reason our brains trick us into thinking we must exercise for an hour a day, seven days a week, inside a gym with fancy equipment. Good news! The last time I checked, you can exercise practically anywhere, without equipment, on your own terms, and for however long you feel like it. What we all need to understand is that exercise is not rocket science. It's easier than we think. If we stop making it out to be the doom, gloom, dark cloud of disgust…we may actually find it enjoyable and stick to it long enough to reap the benefits for the rest of our lives.

If you fall off the fitness bandwagon or are not in the mood today, **TAKE FIVE**. I am not talking about the candy bar, the lotto game, or Dave Brubeck's best-selling album (for those of you into jazz music). I am talking about time. More specifically, I'm talking about **MINUTES**. Take five, consecutive minutes out of your busy day to exercise. It can be anything from dancing in your kitchen to jumping all over Couch to vigorously combing through your hair. Anything that increases your heart rate above what it is when you are sitting on Couch counts. It's a known fact that five minutes of mild exercise makes your heart beat faster and increases oxygen delivery to your muscles. Yay! You can increase your time and eventually work up to those thirty recommended minutes of moderate-intensity exercise, five days per week. But for now, start with five minutes and see how much easier it is to get started. Make yourself and your health a priority for five minutes a day. If you drive to the gym and go on the elliptical for five minutes and walk right back out the door... you've succeeded. Congratulations, you did it! Don't stress yourself out about exercise because exercise is supposed to melt away the stress. The truth is you have five minutes. We all do. Check out the **5 Minute Home Workouts** app for home exercise routines for both men and women.

ONE THING AT A TIME

Karin asked for a six-week exercise program to complete on the days I am not training with her. The fitness plan I came up with consisted of six to seven exercises in a circuit style that would take anywhere from twenty to thirty minutes, depending on the day. When I checked in with Karin at our sessions each Friday, she admitted she was not completing the exercises, even though she had them printed out with descriptions and photos. I asked her why she wasn't completing the workouts on her own. Here was her response: *"I just can't motivate myself to do that much by myself."* She continued, saying that even though it seemed easy and she understood exactly what the exercises were and how to do them, she became overwhelmed and lost her motivation when she went to complete them on her own.

"Was the task really that difficult?" I wondered. As an experiment, I decided to make a simple change. I began to text Karin one exercise each morning. She did not know what each morning's exercise would be in advance. I gave her instructions like, *"Try 20 push-ups. How many sets of those can you do throughout the day today?"* This *one-a-day* focus encouraged her to exercise daily with one hundred percent compliance. To her it was *only* one exercise, which made it easier and appeared less overwhelming. She knew it was only going to take a minute or two at most, which gave her the freedom to decide how many times she could do twenty repetitions during her busy day.

Keeping things simple is truthfully the best way to propel your love of exercise forward. Let's be honest: we are not interested in things that take more effort, more remembering, and more work. Being overwhelmed is not fun, and the brain does not want to work harder than it has to. You can and should increase your effort after the "exercise ball" gets rolling. But in the beginning, if you take just one step at a time, one day at a time, one movement at a time, one exercise at a time, those small changes will add up.

CHAPTER 1

SUMMARY

✓ Start small by focusing on one thing at a time. Do not get overwhelmed and stressed out.

✓ Walk more. It is the simplest way to increase your activity. Get up and get walking.

✓ Fidget, which really means move around more. Little movements throughout your day add up, so don't forget to make the most of your actions.

✓ Take five minutes to start and engage in continuous exercise that increases your heart rate for five consecutive minutes.

✓ Focus on one exercise each day. It does not take much to get you into a healthy habit.

CHAPTER 2

Put It In Writing

"Start writing, no matter what. The water does not flow until the faucet is turned on."
—*Louis L'Amour*

Scarlet was about to scarf down her warm chocolate chip cookie when she glanced over and noticed the spiral bound notebook taunting her on the coffee table. *"Ugh,"* she cursed at the wretched thing. Looking at the cookie, she debated, *"Do I eat this cookie and not write it down, do I put the cookie down, or do I write the blasted cookie and its calories down in that thing?"* Oh, the guilt. Torn, she decided to go for a ten minute walk and come back to the cookie. The walk made her feel so amazing that she didn't actually want the cookie anymore. It didn't taunt her like it had when she felt she wasn't allowed to have it. Scarlet felt awesome and empowered. She ended up losing five pounds that month. How did she do it?

It's crazy to think that writing things down can make us healthier people, but it is absolutely true! In the case of my dear client Scarlet, what happened was that writing in a *"food journal,"* as most would call it, became an eye-opener for her. The best research shows that staring at yourself in the mirror, so to speak, helps you to see who you really are and how you are living. According to a study from Kaiser Permanente's Center for Health Research published in the *American Journal of Preventative Medicine*, keeping a food journal may double your weight loss efforts. Most of us are in denial or are shielding our eyes from the real truth. Let's discover how to write things down. As you start doing this, I am willing to bet that your story of a healthier life will start to unfold right before your very eyes.

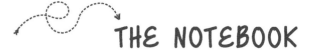

THE NOTEBOOK

When I start any exercise program with my clients, I encourage them to write everything down in a fitness and food journal. Some call it a diary; my male clients tend to call it *"the notebook."* Whatever you name the collection of blank paper or fill-in-the-blanks on the computer screen, it's all the same! Most people are not excited about this process. It is not intended to make anyone feel bad or guilty; it is simply a tool to help you see your habits more clearly. It's a plain ol' reality check. We all need those!

Numerous research studies show that the people who recorded their food intake and logged their exercise were not only more likely to lose weight, but were also able to keep it off longer than those who did not keep track. Journaling your calorie intake (food and fluids), your calorie output (exercise), sleep, and muscle soreness, along with your overall feelings, can be a tool to put you on the road to success. Writing things down builds an awareness of the *what, why,* and *when* of your overall health. It can also help you identify triggers, both physically and emotionally, that you may not have known were there.

In Scarlet's case, she realized after a month of journaling that all she had changed were her habits. It showed her that she liked to eat sweets at night but also that she had time to go for a brisk walk instead of hanging out with Couch. It helped her keep track of her exercise too. If she was sore the next day, she knew exactly why and marked it as a *"love/ hate"* exercise in her book. She didn't always put down the cookie, but instead she monitored when she really, really, really wanted that cookie and when she was just eating out of habit or boredom. Writing things down helps you to see your victories and realize the improvements you need to make. Grab a notebook for the next few weeks, or use the online tools on websites like My Fitness Pal or Spark People, to get started.

A DATE WITH YOURSELF

Why is it that we can keep appointments with others, but we have a hard time keeping appointments with ourselves? If you think about all of the other things you could be doing with those twenty-four precious hours in your day, besides exercise, guess what? You will never have time. You have to make time. Yes, even me. I have to make time too.

People that succeed at sticking to exercise usually schedule it into their day—just like a wedding, hair appointment, or trip to the dentist. Circle your exercise appointment in red on your calendar or, like many people, use an alarm or enter appointments into your phone (hard to forget when you carry it with you all day). Stop giving in to Couch and its slimy ways and put your exercise on the books! You can highlight it, circle it, and put gold stars next to it. Do whatever works to ensure you take action. Try this: For the next two to three days, write down how you spend your time. Afterwards, take a look at what your *"time sucks"* are. In other words, which activities are a complete waste of your time? My *"time suck"*, for example, is folding laundry. Ugh! Where can you squeeze in some exercise instead of engaging in time-sucking activities?

For the next few weeks, I want you to schedule in some exercise time on your actual calendar. Schedule a fitness appointment with yourself and be sure to use permanent marker. If you use electronic calendars, put it in there highlighted or marked in red so it stands out.

Utilize Apps like **Awesome Note 2** and **Pocket Life Calendar**. These are great for keeping your calendar organized and even getting custom alerts.

Try to prohibit yourself from editing, erasing, or rescheduling over and over again. This is a great opportunity to show off your time management skills! After all, you're the boss, and you don't want to have to fire yourself.

LIST IT, DO IT, CHILL OUT!

Make that list, and check it twice. Who's been naughty and who's been nice? To-do lists run my household! I usually write things down or they don't get done. Plus, checking things off of the list makes me feel warm and fuzzy all over. It's that whole feeling-of-accomplishment thing. The same *"to-do"* list concept applies to daily exercise and activity, but I like to call it a TO-DAY list (as in, what kind of activity or exercise would I like to accomplish to-day?).

Emily searched for a workout on the internet and took one brief look before rushing off to the gym. When she got there, she banged through the list and often forgot how many sets or reps the workout said to complete. She would tell me that she had meant to do push-ups, but she forgot once she got to the gym. Hence, the importance of having a physical list! Try not to keep it in your head, but instead actually write it down, or type it into whatever techy device you have. What good is it if you can't remember it? Follow these simple instructions to make your fit to-day list:

✔ First, determine what you would like to accomplish with your exercise today, and be detailed. If it's a five-minute walk, then mark that specific action on your to-day list. Don't just write EXERCISE. Our brain thinks that is too big of a task, especially if we haven't exercised before or are just getting back on the exercise train. Choo Choo!

✔ Start your list with a maximum of three items. If you have more than one exercise or activity (like Emily did), put them in an organized list and try to tackle the most difficult thing first in order to knock it out of the way. This will help you gain momentum for the rest of the workout and help you make progress.

✔ Record the specific amount of sets, weight, and repetitions for each exercise on your list. If you have been to a gym, you might see clients with paper and clipboards keeping track of their exercises and checking them off when they are complete. It's important to have a clear and concise goal for the day and enforce the self-control needed to achieve it. No guessing, no stalling, just doing. Ah, the feeling of accomplishment!

Make that list, and check it twice!

STICK IT TO 'EM

Sticky notes are another staple in my household. For example, posted on the front door is, *"Don't forget to wipe your feet,"* and posted on the bathroom mirror is, *"Don't forget to wash your hands."* Those are mostly for my messy and often forgetful boys! I love them dearly. I have a few sticky notes just for me, though, stuck to my bathroom mirror and on my sneaker rack. Those notes say: *"Today is a brand new day,"* and *"Life is short, get out and have fun."* These are small reminders just for me-my very own slice of daily inspiration.

My client, Jan, placed a sticky note on her refrigerator that says, *"Eat clean so you can sleep well."* Jan is a night eater, so the reminder helps her stay away from those dinner left-overs she used to warm up at 10:00 pm. Every small reminder counts, and each can be the difference between success and failure. The advantage that a sticky note or blank sticky piece of paper offers is that you can write anything on it. Sticky notes allow us to be very specific and drill down to our exact needs.

Let's get going. Write yourself some inspiration today:

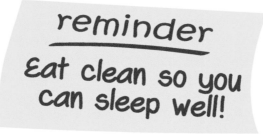

reminder

Eat clean so you can sleep well!

- ☐ Get some sticky notes and a pen. If you don't have sticky notes, use some tape or glue, maple syrup, or already-been-chewed gum. Be creative here! I suggest you keep these notes wherever you will see them numerous times throughout your day, and post them at eye level. This includes your car and your workplace.

- ☐ Get specific, and list the things you are going to start doing to reach your goal and the things you should stop doing to be able to reach your goals. For example, you can post notes all over Couch that say, *"Don't sit on me. Go for a walk!"* Couch loves that one!

- ☐ Hold yourself accountable by posting questions like, *"Did you go for your daily walk today?"*

- ☐ Create challenges such as, *"Think you can make it an extra five minutes on your walks this week?"* Hey, why not try?

- ☐ Make your statements clear, concise, and consistent with what you want to accomplish. Consistency leads to habit.

Healthy habits equal happy people. There are no limits to what a sticky can say—so get writing, and stick them everywhere!

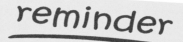

reminder

UPDATE YOUR PROFILE

Alana's husband starts our fitness consultation by telling me Alana has failed miserably in the past with exercise programs. He elaborates by explaining she tried it all: diet fads, supplements, fitness parties, exercise classes, new exercise equipment, QVC *"contraptions"* (as he put it). You name it, she's tried it. I responded, *"You don't know until you try, right? Maybe that spin class just wasn't for her."* The truth of the matter is, you may be down on yourself like Alana was for never sticking with exercise or diet plans. Well, Michael Jordan was passed over for the varsity high school basketball team during his sophomore year. Seriously, if he had stopped there and didn't keep trying, we would never know him as the greatest basketball player of all time. Think about that for a moment. Kind of crazy, isn't it? Others like Abraham Lincoln, Benjamin Franklin, and Helen Keller were in the same boat. These famous icons persevered. If at first you don't succeed, try again, and try something different.

I proceeded to ask Alana what made her good at her job. She was a sales representative for a Fortune 500 company and was in the top ten percent of the sales force. She said, *"I guess I am really great at focusing on the task I need to complete each day. I plan it, I focus on it, and I execute it."* We then discussed how she could apply those skills to her exercise.

I don't care who you are, you have been a raging success at something. We all have different talents and strengths. What are yours? What are you naturally good at?

Try this activity to build self-awareness of your great qualities:

> ☐ **Write down a list of times you were successful at something. It could be anything. No limits here.**
>
> ☐ **In another column, write down how you accomplished those things and why you didn't give up until you succeeded. Why were you so determined? Was someone twisting your arm?**
>
> ☐ **List three qualities about yourself that you value and that make you who you are.**
>
> ☐ **Write down three ways you can use your awesome qualities to apply to your exercise habits.**

Take this piece of paper and reflect on your successes, no matter how big or how small. Remind yourself of the qualities you possess, and apply them to your fitness attitude. Heck, put them on a sticky note while you're at it.

SIGN ON THE DOTTED LINE

Contracts get things done! Any business will tell you this. Just think of a time you signed a contract-it could've been anything from starting the construction of your new house to enrolling your kids in preschool. When you sign and date a contract, it's official. The work can now begin. I tried this with a few of my clients and found that those who wrote and signed a three month contract not only reached their goal, but, in most cases, surpassed it within the three month timeframe. How can this be?

When you write a contract, it mentally encourages you to stick to it. Every day that you adhere to that promise to yourself, it gives you a big, awesome fist pump that, in turn, builds up your confidence that YOU REALLY CAN DO IT. Seeing your goals on paper, signed at the bottom with your name, makes your journey to a healthier lifestyle all the more real. Think of the contract as divorce papers for Couch. Read them and weep!

☐ Start with this simple contract: I, [your full name], will move for five consecutive minutes each day. It can be anytime, anywhere. It can be walking, biking, jogging, hiking, cooking, or anything that gets me off my butt and increases my heart rate. I must do it consistently for five minutes, no matter what. This will help me feel accomplished and proud of my commitment to live a healthier and happier life. I will be proud of myself when my head hits the pillow at night. Start date 01/01/__.

☐ Sign and date your contract in permanent ink. I should mention that having a witness helps. It's the accountability thing again! Having a witness certainly helps with your follow-through.

☐ **Make sure your contract is for the next thirty to ninety days, and it is very specific, including the details of your wants and desires.**

Use online tools like **Beeminder**. This site allows you to sign a contract, report in, and track your own Yellow Brick Road.

When you write a contract, it mentally encourages you to stick to it.

Think of the contract as divorce papers for Couch. Read them and weep!

_____   _____
Name   Date

CHAPTER 2

SUMMARY

- Start by keeping a notebook or *"journal."* This will open your eyes to what is really going on, both physically and mentally.

- Schedule your workouts on your calendar. You don't always have time, so you have to make time.

- Start an exercise To-day list. Whether it is one exercise or a list of exercises, write them down and have them organized in the order you are going to tackle them.

- Post inspirational notes all around where you can see them every day. This will keep you focused and inspired.

- Make a contract with yourself. This provides an official document for you to get started with the plan and ultimately achieve success.

CHAPTER 3

Dump Those Comfy Habits

"Winning is a habit. Unfortunately,
so is losing."
—*Vince Lombardi*

Look at Couch sitting over there with its worn out cushions. Goes to show how much we depended on it. It feels good to know we are busting free from its stronghold. Why have we made a habit of sitting? Sitting, like other habits, is a regular practice that is hard to give up. Such habits have placed us in our comfort zones and on our comfy couches. We all form habits in most of our daily activities. We often call these "routines." Wouldn't it be annoying if you had to think about how you were going to shower every day? First the shampoo, then the soap. Wait-soap first, then the shampoo? Every habit was new once, and you developed it to serve a purpose at some point in time. That kid who picked his nose in second grade may have started to because he was bored in math class. It does not mean he should still be picking his nose, right? Habits must change in order for life to keep moving forward and for us to grow. It is challenging to change and replace habits, but you need to go for it anyway! After all, *we are what we repeatedly do.*

If you have developed habits that are keeping you from exercising then you need to dump them right away and start developing some new, healthier habits. And if you are still picking your nose, that's got to stop, too. Not a healthy habit!

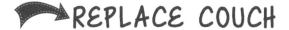REPLACE COUCH

Like an old pair of shoes with worn out soles and patches of discoloration, you need to replace worn out habits with new, fancy, upgraded versions. It is time to say good-bye to things that are making you an old fart! What are you choosing to make your habits? If it involves lying around with Couch all day, you need to ditch it. These lazy and boring actions need to be replaced with exciting and active habits.

An example that comes to mind is that of one of my clients named Jessie. Jessie is a receptionist at a busy office. She does not sit at the front desk but instead, has an office in the back, where she does not have much interaction with customers. She reached out to me for advice. Jessie explained that she couldn't help her sedentary lifestyle because she sits at a desk all day. After a few minutes of conversation, we discussed the option of using a stability ball as her chair instead of the black leather contraption. The stability ball would encourage Jessie to move around while at work but still enable her to perform her daily tasks. She started there and noticed it was easier for her to keep moving throughout her day. Since then, Jessie has purchased a stand up desk and switches from the stability ball to standing throughout her day. The simple act of replacing a *"sit"* habit with a more active, *"fit"* alternative is a great way to get started with a healthier lifestyle.

I want you to think of a habit where you are sitting instead of moving. Can you replace it with a healthier habit? Here are some examples where you can replace Couch with more active habits:

☐ Stand at the counter to eat your snacks.

☐ Go for a walk to return your phone calls during work.

☐ Eat your lunch standing up.

☐ Purchase foot pedals so you can *"bike"* while you sit.

☐ Watch TV while walking using cardio equipment.

☐ Read your books while sitting on a stability ball.

☐ Do jumping jacks while yelling at your kids to clean up!

☐ Pretend you are a rockstar and play some air guitar while dialed into your hour long conference call (don't tell your boss about this one!).

☐ Stand while reading the newspaper.

PICK A TIME

In 1960, Dr. Maxwell Maltz wrote a book called *Psycho Cybernetics* that argued that it takes 21 days to change a habit. However, new research from the Cancer Research UK Health Behaviour Research Centre proposes that it actually takes over two months (sixty-six days) to do so. As new studies are always being conducted, theories and hard data often seem to change—making it hard to know the real story about habit formation. Does the time frame really matter?

My advice is to focus on CONSISTENCY versus time. If you consistently do something, you are more likely to build a habit out of it. If you consistently bite your nails, it will become a habit. This is not because you bit your nails for 21 days; this is simply because you bit them over and over and over again, until you started to bite them for no apparent reason. So the questions are: how do we build healthy habits, and what's it going to take to get there?

One thing you can use to jumpstart a healthy habit of exercising is going to the same place at the same time. Consistency tends to equal success. I am not saying you can never change this, but when you are just getting started, this will help you build the habit. Think about the same guy you've seen at the gym the few times you actually made it there. If you went at the same time, you would most likely notice the same people. In order to be one of those people who have built the exercise habit, you should try these three golden rules to get your habit of exercise going:

- ☐ Allot time that will not be interrupted by necessary routines (putting kids on the bus, cooking dinner, work meetings, or college class schedules, for example).

- ☐ Allot the same time every day. If you have to get up a few minutes earlier, walk during your lunch break at work, or hit the gym before you end your day…go for it!

MUSTER UP SOME WILLPOWER

You will need serious willpower to stroll past Couch and not cuddle back in during the beginning stages of your break-up. Couch will try to sweet-talk you, but don't fall for it. You must become familiar with willpower and learn how to use it to your advantage. This might seem like it could become deep and complicated, but it doesn't need to be.

Willpower is a muscle. You can sculpt it, change it, mold it, tweak it, and condition it. You need to feed it the right stuff. There are some simple ways to use it and not abuse it. Think of a time you bit your tongue (figuratively) when you really wanted to ream someone out. You had to use some serious willpower to do everything in your control **NOT** to rip them a new one! It takes effort, time, and patience to condition the willpower muscle.

Practicing willpower is like practicing any other skill in life. Practice makes you better. Practice helps you grow. Practice involves discipline. When you think of the people you know who are really good at something, why is that? They had an interest or desire and continued to practice it. It may not have started off as passion, but *"forcing yourself to practice is what starts to build self-regulatory strength"* (Charles Duhigg, *The Power of Habit*). If this is true, then we can practice using willpower and gain strength with it.

Here is a quick activity to practice using your willpower muscle. No matter what, ignore Couch all day today. Don't even glance in its direction. Do everything in your power not to sit. When you do this (even when you don't want to!), that is using some serious willpower. You just have to work the muscle and it will grow over time. As I have discovered, the best way to grow your willpower is by making it a habit. It takes time, so don't get discouraged when you are first starting out. Think of activities in your life that require you to use willpower. Practice using it, and watch how it grows. (Cha Cha Cha Chia!). Read *Willpower* by Roy F. Baumesiter or *The Power of Habit* by Charles Duhigg for more interesting information and insight on willpower.

REWARD YOURSELF

Rewards are great, aren't they? Rewarding yourself for making healthy changes reinforces new habits and can motivate. Why not celebrate your success each step of the way? Since we are adults here, we can move past the sparkly star stickers (unless they still motivate you, of course). If rewards make you feel good and keep you motivated, reward away! Try not to involve food rewards, though. Since these undermine your efforts, keep food out of the healthy-lifestyle equation.

Here are some suggestions of ways to celebrate your success:

☐ Splurge, and treat yourself to new fitness attire.

☐ Schedule a 60-minute massage.

☐ Get a fresh hair cut or hairdo.

☐ Dress up and go out on the town.

☐ Spa day—at home or at the salon.

☐ Take a day off of work and schedule something FUN.

☐ Get a new picture on your driver's license.

☐ Get fitted for some new workout shoes at a running store.

☐ Book a consult or session with a personal trainer or dietician.

☐ Schedule a professional photo shoot.

☐ Book a long-weekend vacation doing something active.

Remember to pick rewards that are out of the ordinary, within your budget, and worth achieving. They should be in line with your goals. Reward yourself at certain milestones, and make sure you are writing them down, just as you write down your goals. For example, if your goal is to fit into that little black dress you wore two years ago at your cousin's wedding, perhaps for every half an inch you lose in your waist, you can reward yourself with a new accessory that will make you feel sexy when you get back into that dress. It does not have to be expensive; it can be a new nail polish or hairpin with *bling* on it. Just find what works for you and celebrate. Explore apps like **NexTrack** for rewards associated with the amount of activity you complete.

PLACE YOUR BETS

Another interesting thing about rewards is that we tend to work harder when money is involved. I bet Couch will be really mad at you after hearing this! In fact, the use of money impacts us even more if it is taken away from us, as opposed to awarded to us. Academic research shows that individuals who risk losing some mullah of their own shed more pounds than those who receive no penalty or reward. When you put money into weight loss and exercise contests, you now have some skin in the game, so to speak. It dangles the carrot on one end, but also provides the risk of losing your money on the other end.

Money is tangible and can help us get some extra motivation in the short term and jumpstart the process of getting healthier in the long term. Would you like to try out this theory? The good news is, there's an app for that (and a website, for those of you who prefer computers to complicated phones)!

Gym-Pact: You will be forced to put your money where your exercise is! Commit to a specific number of days per week during which you plan to exercise, and fill in how much you will pay if you don't follow through with your plan. You must check in at your workout location so that the app can locate you via GPS for confirmation. Hello, accountability factor!

HealthyWage: This health-incentives company provides an incentive program tailored to specific goals, like losing weight. You can participate in a team challenge, or make a healthy wager.

stickK: Sign a commitment contract and decide which charity will receive your money if you don't reach your goals. You can also choose *"anti-charities,"* which are specific organizations that you are opposed to. This is meant to provide you with the motivation to not give them any of your cold, hard cash.

21 Habit: This app allows you to invest your money in your commitment, but you will only get your money back if you keep up with your goals. Money you lose to this challenge will be sent to a charity which will keep you honest about your performance.

CHAPTER 3

SUMMARY

✓ Replace a sedentary habit with a moving habit.

✓ Try to exercise at the same time every day. This should be a time that is most convenient for you and one for which you won't have any excuses. Consistency is key.

✓ Practice using your willpower. This will strengthen over time and lead to the habit of exercising.

✓ Reward yourself for reaching milestones along the road to reaching your bigger goals. Prizes and money can help stir up some motivation.

✓ Losing your money can help you break out of those non-healthy habits. Wager some of your hard-earned cash, and it may just help you out of a lazy rut.

CHAPTER 4

Lean On Me

"Alone we can do so little;
together we can do so much."
— *Helen Keller*

Imagine the song *Lean on Me* by Bill Withers playing in the background. Can you hear it? Now, think of the people you lean on for support when you are going through a bad break-up or experience loss. You need those you trust to keep you motivated and moving forward in your journey. Those in your circle of trust are instrumental in keeping you from going back to your old ways or feeling sorry for yourself. People who are successful at leaving Couch behind and moving on to better things usually have a team of people to thank. Think of the speeches given at the Grammys, the Oscars, or the Super Bowl. Many start with, *"I want to thank God,"* followed by a long list of people we may or may not have heard of. There are always the behind-the-scenes people who can make or break your success. What would Ellen DeGeneres be without her sound guy? What would *Saturday Night Live* be without its writers? I couldn't have published this book without my editors, my photographer, my graphic designer, my formatter, my cover designer, and the strong support of my friends and family. In life, we all just need someone to lean on and reach out to when we need help.

Consider what Roy F. Baumeister and John Tierney describe in their book *Willpower* as the *"Oprah Paradox."* Oprah has had a few ups and downs in her weight-loss efforts. When she was successful at losing the weight, she attributed it to a personal trainer, a chef, a nutritionist, a counselor, and many personal assistants. Baumeister explains that a team of experts was necessary in Oprah's case because she used up her willpower in other areas of her life and work. When it came to exercise, her willpower was depleted, and so she needed to call in the big dogs. If you get what you need by calling in the reinforcements, then why not? Why not employ people who can help you reach your goals? If you can't kick your own keister, hire someone to do it for you! It's **OK** to admit you need professional help. It's **OK** to hire a team of help. It may be all it takes to give you a good jumpstart into exercise.

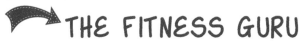

THE FITNESS GURU

When I first met Karla, she said right off the bat, *"I will not respond well if you yell at me."* As we continued with our conversation, she got to know me better and discovered that it is not my style to *"yell"* at my clients. I told her that I would be there to encourage her, but that it was not my nature to do so by yelling like an Army drill sergeant. It was a great start to our consult because Karla was being crystal clear about her needs. It revealed her personality and helped me to determine if we would be a good fit.

Sometimes you know what you should be doing, but you need someone there to motivate you to actually do it. With my business in particular, I travel to people's homes and offices to assist them with their exercise program. It's hard to turn your lights off and pretend you are not home when I am standing on your front porch. You can try to hide, but I know you're in there!

People hire personal trainers for many reasons, but motivation and guidance are the biggest need for most. You may need answers to questions like: what weights do I lift? how many reps do I complete? what types of exercises should I be doing? You may need or want a fitness buddy, perhaps someone to hold you accountable and/or a person who will challenge you. This is what good trainers live for!

In order to choose a trainer, you need to do your research and, like Karla, clearly communicate your wants and needs. Not all trainers offer the same level of expertise and certainly do not have the same training style. This is a good thing though. Differences make the world go round.

Here are some quick tips on what you should look for in a personal trainer and how you can benefit from hiring one:

>> **Personality:** You want to make sure you find a trainer who fits your personality. Otherwise, this could go south real fast! Ask questions like, *"What is your style of training?"* or *"How do you motivate your clients?"* This will tell you a lot.

>> **Certifications:** You should make sure the personal trainer has acquired their certification through a nationally accredited agency. This is important for injury prevention. Look for the NCCA accreditation. This is a third-party-certifying organization.

>> **Fitness Assessment:** Your trainer should talk to you about your goals and complete a fitness assessment with you. If you meet your trainer on day one and start working out right away, that's a big red flag! It's not enough time for the trainer to thoroughly study and assess your detailed health information. If they care, they will take time to review it.

>> **Undivided Attention:** Your trainer should not be texting, emailing, or answering other calls when they are with you. You are paying for that time, and it is important that they commit to you as a person and shows genuine interest in helping you achieve and exceed your goals.

>> **Adjustments:** Your trainer should change up the program every couple of months. Every fitness program should provide tweaks and progressions. If you are always doing the same things, your results are always going to be the same.

>> **Motivation:** Your trainer is there to motivate you, cheer you on, inspire you to be more, make sure you don't get injured, educate you, and support you. If you are not *feeling the love,*

then it's not a good fit. You should look forward to seeing this person, and they should always ensure that you leave your workout satisfied and proud of yourself.

To find a reputable Certified Personal Trainer in your area, visit ideafit.com. Just enter your zip code, and explore trainers' profiles, credentials, experience, client reviews and more. If you like the idea of one-on-one training but are more interested in online training and videos, you may like the app **Wello**. This app lets you pick a space to exercise in, along with your specific activity interest, and the app will find you available trainers. Niketrainingclub.com also offers online personal trainers, workouts, and training advice. Self.com is another great resource full of advice and training from the pros that know.

TALK IT OVER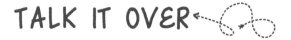

Mallory and I met on and off for two years. She had a sales job, so she traveled in the car all day, and she would dine out with clients during the evenings. She gained a significant amount of weight and needed to lose it for various health reasons. We tried outdoor workouts at the park, meeting at the gym, and exercising in her house. She always put work and her family first. This led to many cancellations and "holds" on our training programs. I received texts like, *"I am just too tired today,"* or *"I have a conference call I forgot about,"* or *"Let's start back up in September."* The last time I reached out to her after months of not meeting, she let me know that she finally decided to see a therapist and was getting her mind in a good place.

Mallory was proud to tell me she was now walking every day and had incorporated healthy foods into her diet. I commended her for finding the person she needed to move things along, for good. It was important for her to realize that she didn't have to start with a personal trainer, but instead, explore other options.

This is what professional therapists are for! They are trained and educated in diagnosing and treating mental, emotional, and behavioral disorders. Knowing what you need help with and putting those experts in your path is one of the smartest moves you can make. I feel like a therapist sometimes. I do not, however, hold a degree in psychology, and some problems go deeper than I can or should handle. This is what the professional therapists and life coaches are for! They are educated about the psychology of what motivates you specifically. It is all about YOU. We are all different, so knowing this is half the battle.

Deep discussions are are usually necessary to spark change. They bring out the root cause of many issues and sometimes we can't even get out of our own way to see what those are. It never hurts to talk with someone who can give you professional guidance and their non-biased listening ear. Wellness coaches, life coaches, and behavioral psychologists are all what you should be searching for if you are interested in making mindset changes but don't know where to start.

Just as with a personal trainer, the price point of these professionals can run the gamut. No matter the cost, you must ask yourself how much you are willing to invest in your well-being. It can be difficult to know what to search for but typically most of these experts have titles such as therapist, counselor, or coach.

Start with these suggestions, and hopefully you will be better able to narrow things down:

>> **ASK** your insurance company for help. They will have a list of providers in your area and will let you know which ones are covered by your insurance plan.

>> **ASK** your employer. They may have assistance programs that can lead you in the right direction.

>> **ASK** a friend who already has a therapist for a recommendation. If your friend often raves about their therapist, ask them for contact information.

>> **VISIT** the **Psychology Today** website, an online resource that answers a ton of questions about what to look for in a therapist. This site will even help you find some local providers in your area when you input your zip code.

>> **TRY** the **Talkspace** app for minor stressors and a sounding board with email exchanges, therapy and counseling.

>> **TRY** the **Tumbtack** app. This app allows you to be specific and enter exactly what you need. Qualified candidates in your area will pop up and you can choose the one that feels right for you even according to your budget.

THE PERFECT RECIPE

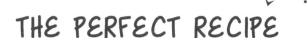

OK, so here is the deal with food. Food is fuel. As Tony Horton puts it, *"Food is health and exercise is fitness."* Without the proper nutrients to fuel the muscles you are working to strengthen, you will not see the changes you desire. For example, consider that your low self-control or willpower might be caused by a low glucose level. Consider that your lack of motivation might be caused by not drinking enough water. You need half of your body weight in ounces per day. Are you getting that?

If you are not eating the proper nutrients before your workouts, you may not have the gusto you need at the gym in order to push through your routine. If you are not eating the proper combination of nutrients after, you may not be maximizing your gains and helping your body recover from exercise. Diet and exercise **MUST** go together. They are the perfect pair. This is why it is very important to get advice and expertise from the right professionals.

According to the American Dietetic Association, most states have statutes that regulate or license nutritionists. A registered dietician has an R.D. in their title and holds a four-year degree in nutrition and dietetics. Although I do not want to discount other certifications (after all, I know an exorbitant amount of information about nutrition and have completed a specialized certification as a weight loss specialist), registered dietitians should be the experts creating specific menus plans, recommending supplements, and selecting recipes for you. I highly suggest talking to a registered dietician if you have been struggling with weight loss, have no idea what to eat or where to start, have food allergies or sensitivities, have a disease, have high cholesterol, have certain digestive disorders, or have had gastric surgery (just to name a few). If you are looking to go the au naturel route, there are also some holistic nutritionists with years of study and experience who may be good options as well. Check out your local Chamber of Commerce for recommended dieticians in your area. For those of you who want to hire a R. D. N. from behind closed doors and keep them in your pocket, try an app like **Rise**. This is a great option for those who want advice on making daily dietary decisions and some hand-holding as well. If you are just searching for a simple place to start, be sure to visit www. choosemyplate.gov for guidelines, recipes, charts, and various nutritional information. No matter which direction you go, make sure you trust the person and the source.

CHAPTER 4

SUMMARY

- Find a team full of people that will support, inspire, and help you reach your mission in life.

- Hire a personal trainer if you need help with exercise program ideas, guidance, and motivation. They can be your best fitness buddy.

- Hire a life coach or therapist if you need help with your all-around lifestyle, attitude, or past experiences which might be hindering your progress toward a fit and healthy lifestyle. Sometimes it may be deeper rooted than we are even aware of.

- Hire a registered dietician if you feel that food and lack of education about dietary needs may be part of your issue. A dietician's expertise may be just the sort of guidance you need to be on your way.

CHAPTER 5

Gathering Up Your Things

"Start where you are. Use what you have.
Do what you can."
—Arthur Ash

When you are walking around with your cardboard box gathering up your things, you are going to need some extra tools to leave Couch for good. What you choose to take with you makes all the difference. One of the lessons I like to teach my children is to use their resources. I become easily annoyed when they tell me they can't do their homework because they don't have a ruler or know how to spell a word. I ask them, *"What would you do if I was not here? You would use a dictionary, right?" "You would find a ruler on the internet and print it out."* When you learn to use your resources wisely, you find ways to get answers. It may take extra effort, but I promise you that resourcefulness will help you to achieve the end result of moving on from your sedentary ways. Using the right resources encourages you to think outside the box to get things done. Nice to meet you, creativity!

The same goes for the exercise world. There are resources all around you. Endless books, websites, videos, magazines, articles, podcasts, classes, webinars, seminars, free events, etc. I agree it can be overwhelming and that sometimes there are so many choices we don't know how to narrow them down. Do I start with 30 days? Do I go short and sweet? Do I change my diet first and then exercise? If you are not able to hire a personal trainer, nutritionist, or therapist (as discussed in the last chapter) but want to try becoming more active and informed on your own first, this chapter is for you. I will provide some specific ideas on how to use books, magazines, DVDs, and other great resources to help you get started on your fitness journey.

PICK FROM THE MAGAZINE RACK

Everyone has a story. Have you ever gone to a conference where you've heard someone tell their story, and you can relate? You think to yourself (or say out loud), AMEN! Someone knows what you have been talking about or has experienced what you are going through. That's because you are not alone, especially when it comes to exercise and lack of motivation. I challenge you to pick up a magazine like *Self, Fitness, Real Simple, Oxygen, Men's Health, People, Women's Health,* or *Prevention* to name a few. These magazines usually have a slew of success stories in each issue. Thumb through them in the store and pick a story you relate to. Are you the single mom working full time to feed three children who barely has enough time to use the bathroom—let alone exercise? Are you the emotional eater who can't seem to break the habit? Are you a workaholic who puts business before yourself…always? Find the story and think to yourself, *"If they can do it, so can I."* Stories can be a big motivator for some people. That is exactly why the magazine publishers continue to feature success stories. It's nice to know you are not alone in your struggles and to learn how people in similar situations did it. It gives you hope and inspiration. Let's find your story:

☐ Look for a magazine that you are interested in that also contains a few success stories.

☐ Tear out the story (after you've bought the magazine or made a copy!) you relate to most and highlight one thing you liked or that you think you may be able to try from another's story. It will help you realize that others like you have succeeded and that you are no different from them. Why not you?

☐ Now that you have an example of what speaks to you, try writing your own success story, outline, or even a bulleted list. Imagine that the editor of the magazine called for people to submit their stories of success and that ten entries will be featured in next month's issue. You could be famous! Think about what you would want everyone to know and which parts of your story you'd want to share to inspire others.

☐ Hang the story up next to your goals and work on making it a reality. Someday, you may get the chance to share your story and be a true inspiration to someone struggling the same way you were.

GRAB THE VIDEOS

I have worked with Anna for over a year now. We have done everything from step aerobics to martial arts! She willingly tried all the workouts I brought and quickly determined which ones were her favorites and which ones she'd prefer to live without. We used a music playlist to get into our workout, whatever it was for that day. On the days we were not training together, she tried to get on the elliptical or the treadmill but found that she was bored and simply going through the motions. She was not motivated to exercise without me.

My suggestion to her was to try an exercise DVD. At first Anna was hesitant; she thought it might be boring and, as she put it, *"Those people in those videos are always so cheesy."*

After she decided to finally take my suggestion, she strolled up and down the exercise section at a local department store and found a Just Dance DVD. To her surprise, she loved it—and so did her daughter. Anna and her daughter danced a few nights a week after her daughter got off of the school bus. It was a fun time they looked forward to. They both burned calories without even knowing it!

Have you ever purchased an exercise DVD or utilized YouTube (it's FREE) for exercise videos? What did you like? What didn't you like? Any department store sells exercise videos in either the sporting goods or movie sections. I challenge you to take a glance around the aisles. You can also find some of the exercise channels offered on cable television that seem interesting or fun to you. If you have never tried any of these suggestions, branch out and give it a go. If you are more of a homebody, you can also complete a Google search for *"exercise DVDs for beginners."* There are many choices: dance, cardio, strength, yoga, kettlebells, ballet, kickboxing, weight training, prenatal, Pilates…you name it. The investment is minimal, and you may actually find something you love. Get to the store, visit the web, or shop online to see what you can find.

THROW IN A FEW GOOD BOOKS

Usually, exercise books have a ripped, sweaty guy flexing his biceps at you or an oiled up hottie in a sports bra giving the skinny arm pose. Though they look great, you may think, *"This is not the book for me."* My advice is that if you are just a beginner to exercise, you do not need to look at the books that give you the scientific details about exercise (unless the details interest you, of course). What you really need is to start small and focus on one element.

This may sound surprising to you, but I don't encourage people to start with exercise or fitness books. Most of the time a self-help book is a better start. Maybe you lack confidence and that's what is holding you back from kicking Couch to the curb. Perhaps you are an avid procrastinator and need to work on that first so that you don't procrastinate on your workouts, too. Often times these types of books will inspire us and teach us new ways of changing old behaviors that get in our way. Some books I suggest are:

- *The Slight Edge* by Jeff Olsen
- *You are Badass* by Jenn Sincero
- *Think and Grow Rich* by Napoleon Hill
- *Unlimited Power* by Tony Robbins
- *The 7 Habits of Highly Effective People* by Stephen Covey
- *The Power of Habit* by Charles Duhigg
- *Who Moved My Cheese?* by Dr. Spencer Johnson
- *Believe and Achieve* by W. Clement Stone
- *Life is Short—Wear Your Party Pants* by Loretta LaRoche

- *Sacred success* by Barbara Stanny
- *Get Out of Your Own Way* by Robert K. Cooper
- *Tools of Titans* by Tim Ferriss

One important point is that most of these books are also available as audiobooks. If you are a book lover, try downloading a book or podcast and walk while listening instead of sitting on Couch to read it. Take your reading time each day, and use that as your exercise time as well. You can kill two Couches with one walk! Download something you are interested in listening to (podcasts are an option here too), and lace up your sneakers. You're going out!

CHAPTER 5

SUMMARY

- ✓ Use available media, multimedia, and printed materials to assist you with beginning to make exercise a part of your life.

- ✓ Use magazines: find a success story that you can relate to, and picture yourself reaching your goals. Write your own success story.

- ✓ Videos and exercise DVDs can offer a whole new world of possibilities. Try some new ones, and see what you think.

- ✓ Make sure to build your library with self-help and motivational books. This not only builds inspiration but helps with all aspects of self-awareness.

CHAPTER 6

Face the Ups and Downs

"When the winds of change blow, some build walls and others build windmills."
—**Chinese Proverb**

Every breakup has stages of healing. You start by weighing the pros and cons. One day you may feel like you've made the best decision of your life to leave Couch, but the next, you may be second-guessing yourself. Dealing with setbacks and obstacles are part of the journey. There will be storms, but they are just passing through. Allow yourself to feel the emotions. They will help propel you forward to a place of confidence and rebirth. Unwanted circumstances and negativity creep up on all of us. It takes work to send those negative vibes running for the hills. Everything has energy, so pick the people, events, and experiences that lift you up and don't bring you down. It will make a world of difference.

This chapter addresses the good, the bad, and the ugly—and how to embrace them all. I have said it before, and I will say it again: this is real life. We must learn to roll with the punches and bend, but not break. Exercise and our ability to keep it as a priority in our lives is much more a mental (or emotional) battle than a physical one. If you approach a healthy lifestyle and exercise in a new, positive light, you may actually start and continue to enjoy it. Read on and you will see how to transform your attitudes and outlooks. The rest is sure to follow and will leave Couch feeling all alone.

AFFIRM THE POSITIVE

Surround yourself with positive people, especially during a breakup. We have all heard the saying, *"Birds of a feather flock together."* Why do you think this is? It's mostly common sense, but as The Law of Attraction states, *"Like attracts like."* If you are negative, you will attract negative things and people to you. Everything and everyone has energy with a certain frequency attached to them. Which would you rather have? It's a simple concept that has been around for centuries. In the book *Think and Grow Rich*, author Napoleon Hills suggests that you receive what you constantly think about. If you think, *"I have no idea how to exercise. That's way too hard for me. I don't have the time,"* then you will receive exactly those things. As my editor put in her side-note to me, *"Tsk Tsk. The defeatist attitude!"* If you don't believe me, just try it! You will get what you constantly focus on, no doubt.

You may think you could never be passionate about exercise, but that can change with a minor attitude adjustment. *"Believe and achieve;"* or, as a successful Mary Kay director and client of mine once told me, *"Fake it until you make it."* Think positively about exercise even if you have to fake it in the beginning, and talk about activity in a positive light. If you start talking about positive experiences at the gym or your enjoyment of your new activities, you will start to believe it and even be surprised to find that exercise has become a positive part of your life.

Positive affirmations are a great way to start your day off on the right foot. Stop reliving the memories of you and Couch by using these positive suggestions:

□ Visit **www.everydayaffirmations.org**. They have free, daily affirmations for all sorts of categories: success, prosperity, women, kids, weight loss, exercise, you name it!

□ Utilize free apps like **Unique Daily Affirmations** or **Happify**. These tools and games will help to start your day off on the positive note.

□ Purchase a calendar with a cute little animal doing something silly that will make you smile and keep your day going in the right direction.

□ Actively go in search of positive people, pictures, or quotes. It's easy enough. If you seek, you shall find. And if these suggestions don't work, the books listed in Chapter Five can help (*You are Badass* by Jen Sincero is my personal favorite.)

TAKE INITIATIVE

We are the only ones responsible for our lives (after God, that is.) What we get is a combination of our behavior and our decisions. The *"I can't"* excuse is not valid. I am often known for telling my boys and my clients, *"The only thing you can't do is walk on water and fly. Everything else is doable."* It's perspective, an attitude, a point of view. A person with no legs will tell me they can't exercise. Well, maybe not with your legs, but you can use your arms. I have a client named Carol who suffered a tragic accident and became paralyzed years ago. That hasn't stopped her. She continues to exercise with the goal of getting into her stand-up wheelchair someday soon. When I hear *"I can't"* from others, I tell them to go see Carol, and she will show them how it's done!

Another inspiring story that I often cling to is that of Kyle Maynard. He was born with a rare condition called congenital amputation, which prevents the development of fetal limbs. Though the odds were stacked against him, he did everything in his power to make it to the top, not only in sports, but in life. He became a top wrestler in his high school. Kyle was awarded GNC's World Strongest Teen, and he went on to receive the ESPN Espy award for Best Athlete with a Disability in 2004. Recently in 2014, Maynard became the first quadruple amputee to climb Mount Kilimanjaro WITHOUT ASSISTANCE! His story is absolutely amazing. Check out Kyle Maynard and his entire story on YouTube. My point with each story is that you have to go out and get what you want. Find a way to make it happen. Things are not going to be handed to you.

In the book *The 7 Habits of Highly Effective People*, Steven Covey describes positivity in the proactive model. He explains that we all have the initiative and ability to make things happen. He states, *"Look at the word response ability—the ability to choose your response."* No blame is placed on conditions or circumstances, but behavior, instead, is a product of our own conscious choice. Being proactive means taking charge of your attitude. Choosing to go for a walk instead of sitting on Couch, now that's being proactive! Proactive people take a look at the storm clouds and go for their scheduled run indoors instead. Reactive people say, *"Look at the weather. It's not my fault that I can't go for a run today."* Proactivity helps you build a habit. After all, the word proactive has the word *"active"* in it, for goodness sake! If you want to build a habit of exercising, you have to be proactive about it.

Things will always come up and take over your day. Act on things that will make you grow, and push through obstacles in your path to success. Don't let the environment or other circumstances get in your way. Grab life by the horns, and get going! Your behavior is a reflection of your conscious choices. You will choose to exercise or to snuggle with Couch. It's your free choice. What will you choose?

EMBRACE THE DOWNPOURS

What happens when someone else rains on your parade? As we all know, there will be "Negative Neds" and "Debbie Downers" out there. Call them what you will, but these are people who always seem to complain and whine about life in general. Sometimes these people tear you down and convince you that you can't or won't do something. I bet we all have one or two of these people in our lives. My advice is to spin it around, and let them and their comments fuel your fire.

One Sunday morning, I got a text from my client, Jane, who hates running. The text says, *"I need you to train me for a warrior dash."* For those of you who don't know, a warrior dash is a race comprised of various obstacles, including a course filled with mud, walls to climb over, and tunnels to crawl through. Perplexed, I gave her a call. *"What's up?"* I asked her. *"Shouldn't you start with a 5k and work your way up from there?"* She said, *"Oh, well my husband is going to participate in the race and he said to me, 'You could never run this.'"* Jane said, "Now, it's on." She started training and hurt her knee a few weeks into it. That did not stop her. She ran that race and many others after that. My point is that all she needed to hear was, *"You can't,"* and everything changed. Although her new outlook could be due, in part, to her competitive nature shining through, it is important to note that it was the negativity spurred from her husband that made her say, *"Watch me."*

Just imagine someone telling you that you won't stick to

exercise. You've tried it in the past with numerous diets, gizmos, gym memberships, aerobic classes, treadmill purchases, etc. and you are right back where you started. In case you haven't noticed, you are in control of the **NOW**. If you use circumstances, negative people, or discouraging comments as motivators, you will charge forward and obliterate every little thing that tries to get in your path. Let there be a thunderstorm on your fitness parade. Dance away in the puddles with a smile and whistle a sweet tune in the rain. These are the winds of change coming, and you should let them take hold of you.

MAKE TIME FOR A GOOD CRY

If you feel like you have tried everything and you just can't shake off your negative, depressed attitude, try scheduling a time for your yuckiness! Negative circumstances happen. A toothache, a breakup, the death of a loved one, an injury, an *"I've lost my house keys during a hailstorm"*...it happens. Life is not always full of sunshine and lollipops (though I do love that song). That is why being positive takes work. It feels good to scream into a pillow and shed some tears from time to time. Sometimes going on a tirade with a best bud is all you need. We all know the feeling of getting something off of our chests—and we automatically feel better. Whether you have feelings of guilt, anger, depression, or downright negativity, we sometimes just have that deep-down desire to be grumpy. This is where scheduling time for negativity can be a useful tool. If there is something that happens in your day and you just can't shake it off, schedule a time during which you can share it or dwell on it, either by yourself or with someone who will listen. Do not let your attitude ruin your whole day. Giving yourself permission to spend some time on the particular circumstance or feeling at a later time may help.

This simple, effective activity has helped my family (especially my youngest son, Luke), along with countless others, and I want you to try it:

- ☐ Share your negative feelings with your spouse or close friends, and write it on a piece of paper.

- ☐ Spend no longer than five minutes on your negativity, in conversation or in thought. Set the timer to make sure you don't continue to dwell on it for longer than five minutes.

- ☐ End the conversation and burn that piece of paper. By doing this, you acknowledge your emotions but do not give them power. Burning the paper will put closure on the negativity so that now you can move on, let it go, and start brand new. Let Couch smell those singes! (I should mention that you should burn this negativity in the sink or have water nearby. Safety first!)

CHAPTER 6

SUMMARY

✔ Use positive affirmations daily to keep your attitude and mind in a good place.

✔ Focus on being proactive. Don't let circumstances run you. Instead, roll with the punches no matter what the circumstances, and have a backup plan when life gets in the way.

✔ Use negativity to motivate and fuel your fire. People and circumstances can rain on your parade, but go ahead and let them. Use that energy to get you going.

✔ Schedule a specific time for negativity. Acknowledge it, talk about it, and then let it go.

PART 2

Staying Motivated

Searching For New Love

CHAPTER 7

It's Not You, It's Me

"Be yourself.
Everyone else is already taken."
—Oscar Wilde

Why are you breaking up with Couch? If it asked you, what would you say? Why is exercise and activity important to you? Your answer to *"Why?"* is a little thing I like to call your true motivation. Motivation is what keeps us moving toward our dreams and aspirations. Let's be honest, we all know how it could go: you go on vacation and when you get back, those few missed workouts turn into a few months of missed workouts, and suddenly, you are wondering what the heck happened to you and why you can't do a sit-up to save your life! Motivation can be a tricky thing. Falling out of routine may start the snowball of disaster. It's not about being motivated to exercise all of the time; it's about being motivated when you need to be in order to reach your goals. It's hard to find that internal motivation, especially when Couch is right over there giving us the sad eyes. We don't have to look under a rock to find it though.

Sometimes we don't know what it is that motivates us. In order to find out, we need to uncover the why behind the why. Scientists, psychologists, behavioral therapists, and other experts have been studying this for centuries. If I ask one hundred different people (and I have), *"What motivates you to exercise every day?"* I will get one hundred unique answers. Some may be similar, but we are all different, amazing specimens. There is no such thing as "normal"—and even though there are patterns, we are never going to be motivated by the exact same thing. This is why there are so many suggestions in this book. Pick one or a few that make you hopeful, and try them out. There is no right or wrong. There is just try. Here are tricks to get that sweaty mojo back!

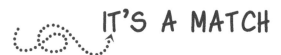

IT'S A MATCH

When I speak to an audience or present at a seminar on fitness and motivation, I start by asking people to think back to when they were young children. I ask these four questions:

- ☐ **What were your favorite things to do when you were little?**
- ☐ **What would you do all day if your parents let you?**
- ☐ **Did you prefer activities with friends or by yourself?**
- ☐ **When people think of you, how would they describe you using only one word?**

I ask them to write a list of answers to each of these questions, and then sit back in their seats and find a common theme. There appear to be three types of fitness personality. Social, antisocial, and go-with-the-flow people. All of your likes and dislikes from your childhood and young-adult lives follow you into future years. It is a reflection of who you are and what your real internal motivational drive will be.

Finding the exercise that works for you is not one-dimensional. As Suzanne Brue, a researcher, writer, and consultant on the connection between personality and physical exercise points out, *"Motivation to exercise can be complex and may include components such as culture, family, friends, finances, and health."* In other words, even training different personality types should be approached with a different pizzazz. You must determine your own personality type in order to find the long-term plan that will work for you.

I am not going to reinvent the wheel here-in order to figure out your fitness personality type, you can use any of the abundant fitness personality quizzes on social media and all over the web. They all give suggestions as to what workouts and styles you should be trying out, as well as ways in which you can play into the strengths of your own personality.

Determining your own personality type will help you find the long-term plan that will work for you.

☐ Try asking yourself this question: Are you a social, antisocial, or go-with-the-flow personality type?

 ☐ Take a few of my favorite fitness personality quizzes found at: **www.bodybuilding.com** and **www.the8colorsoffitness.com** to see if your results match your personality.

☐ When you get the result, be open and try some of the suggestions from the quiz experts. You may find what you've been looking for all along.

☐ If you want to dig a little deeper, read *the 8 colors of fitness* by Suzanne Brue and answer her series of questions (based on the *Myers-Briggs Type Indicator*) about your own personality type.

KISS EXCUSES GOODBYE

Boy, where do we begin with this one? Dr. Wayne W. Dyer explains in his book *Excuses Begone!* that *"Excuses aren't just words explaining the lack of success in various areas of your life-they also show up as pictures or visions that you carry around with you, a series of photos that you see projected on your inner screen."* Sometimes we have used the same excuses for so long that they become our reality. We don't even realize that they are a bunch of lies and avoidance techniques.

Ask yourself, "Why am I making excuses?" We all may think we have valid reasons but really, what is it about exercise that we are trying to avoid? Fear or failure? Lack of results? Trying something new scares us? No matter the excuse, it's about time we throw them away and move forward.

Here is a list of common excuses and why they never work (**P.S.**: This may be harsh, but as Benjamin Franklin put it, *"He that is good for making excuses is seldom good for anything else."*):

≫ I DON'T HAVE TIME—The entire world is busy. It's not just you. No one ever *has* the time; you have to *make* the time.

≫ I AM TOO TIRED—You're tired because you don't exercise. Unless you're sick as a dog with a fever and chills, you have enough energy to exercise. Get up, and get moving.

≫ I AM BORED—Stop doing the same things. You're bored because you are doing boring things. Branch out; be exciting.

≫ THE WEATHER IS BAD—God controls the weather, not us. Embrace the elements, or make a back-up plan and exercise indoors.

≫ I DON'T HAVE A WORKOUT BUDDY—Ask the trainer at the gym if they know anyone who is looking for a fitness pal or ask a co-worker. Visit websites like www.fitnessmeetup.com and www.exercisefriends.com to find a fitness friend in your area that has the same interests and goals as you do.

» **I HAVE KIDS**—Embrace parenthood by being active with your kids. Lead by example. MOVE!

» **I'M TOO OLD**—*"It's not how old you are…it is how you are, 'old'."* You are not old, you just feel it. Go for a walk.

» **I HATE THE GYM**—So don't go to the gym. Exercise can be done anywhere. Nice try.

» **I'M THIN ALREADY**—Umm, NO. Thin does not mean healthy. Try again.

» **I CAN'T AFFORD IT**—Well, exercise is FREE you know. Go to the library, find a book, visit YouTube. Do exercises at home or join a rec league. I am not "buying" this excuse.

» **I CAN'T GET TO THE GYM**—There are trainers out there (ahem…me!) that will travel right to your house.

If you are having a hard time with excuses, it's because you still haven't found something you enjoy. *Excuses Begone!* by Wayne Dyer will help. It's available in audiobook as well. Kiss Couch good-bye and get moving, honey!

LOOK BACK TO MOVE FORWARD

I have a client, Hannah, who hired me in August. It was the hottest part of summer in upstate New York. I told her we would *"walk and talk"* to get to know each other and discuss her fitness goals in detail. Hannah decided to pick a hill by her house. The hill was a gradual, long hill, about one mile in total, but half of the hill was pitched fairly steep. She had told me on the phone that she had been extremely sedentary, had asthma, was very overweight, and suffered from a long list of allergies. One of those allergies happened to be to freshly cut grass, which would induce severe coughing when encountered. Unfortunately, we found that a golf course was at the top of the hill and in the middle of being mowed that day!

Hannah stopped every few steps to bend over, spit on the asphalt, and take a break to catch her breath. She complained of back pain and knee pain. She coughed the entire way and was so red in the face that it made me nervous. It took us an hour, and she could barely talk to me about anything. Feeling discouraged at the end, she said to me, *"That was so hard. I can never do that again."* We named that hill "The Hill of Doom." In the coming weeks, Hannah tackled the hill in bits and pieces. Eventually, she walked the hill at least once a week.

Fast forward one year, and we walked the same hill. Not only did she finish the hill in less than half the time, but she did not spit or cough once (and they were still mowing that darn grass.) She did not complain of knee or back pain at all. We talked the entire time, and she was not out of breath. It was a pinnacle moment for her to see how far she had come in the past year.

- ☐ Take a moment today to reflect on the past and give yourself a pat on the back for how far you have come. Moving further away from Couch takes time, but you are doing it!

- ☐ Picture those riveting moments, and continue moving forward on your journey.

- ☐ Write down the dates of those moments of triumph. Only look back when you want to reflect on your awesomeness! Go and take pictures of the things you have achieved.

reminder

What was once "The Hill of Doom" is now the "Mountain of Achievement."

CHAPTER 7

SUMMARY

- ✓ Find your fitness personality. Take a few quizzes to help you out. It may open your eyes to what you like.

- ✓ Stop making excuses, and start exercising already.

- ✓ Reflect on how far you have come or even how you have found success in the past.

CHAPTER 8

Take Action

*"Setting goals is the first step in turning
the invisible into the visible."*
—*Tony Robbins*

You must continue to increase distance between you and Couch in order to discover your true greatness. Couch has been holding you back all along. Consider the parable of the Old Man on the Hilltop: *"High on a hilltop overlooking the beautiful city of Venice, Italy, there lived an old man who was a genius. Legend had it he could answer any question anyone might ask of him. Two local boys figured they could fool the old man, so they caught a small bird and headed for his residence. One of the boys held the little bird in his hands and asked the old man if the bird was dead or alive. Without hesitation the old man said, 'Son, if I say to you the bird is alive, you will close your hands and crush him to death. If I say the bird is dead, you will open your hands and he will fly away. You see, son, in your hands you hold the power of life and death.'"*

This parable teaches us that we hold the seeds of failure or the potential for greatness. *"Your hands are capable, but they must be used—and for the right things—to reap the rewards you are capable of attaining"* (Frank Purdy: www.goal-setting-for-success.com).

Top executives, athletes, and leaders in all fields set goals. People who are successful in many aspects of their lives tend to be certain about what they want. Creating goals is one way to ensure success. Goals put into perspective what we desire and what we need to do to make desires become reality. Clarifying your goals allows you to live a life with purpose. Goal setting is also important because it helps you organize your time—a valuable asset we wish we had more of. Brian Tracy states in his book *Goals*, *"I have found, over and over, that a person of average intelligence with clear goals will run circles around a genius who is not sure what he or she really wants."* Planning for your more active self is a goal, so let's set some goals and then kick 'em in the face!

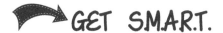 GET S.M.A.R.T.

How are you going to leave Couch for good if you don't know what to do next? It's like saying you are going on a diet, but having no idea what you are going to eat or why you are dieting in the first place. There is an acronym we use to define our goals. I learned this during my years of sales training, but these S.M.A.R.T. goals are out there in all facets of life and not just sales training classrooms. A S.M.A.R.T. goal is a way of breaking down a goal into something we can actually achieve. The S.M.A.R.T. mnemonic stands for:

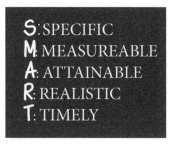

S: SPECIFIC
M: MEASUREABLE
A: ATTAINABLE
R: REALISTIC
T: TIMELY

An example using the mnemonic above would be, *"My goal is to walk for five minutes each evening after dinner. I will do this every day for the next thirty days."* After you write your goal, ask yourself: is this goal specific, measureable, attainable, realistic, and timely? If the answer to all of these questions is, YES, then it is a great goal. It is always OK to reach, readjust, and tweak goals. For example, if someone finds that it is not realistic to commit to a goal on Sundays (but every other day works), then they can change the goal to be attainable and realistic. You want to make the goal challenging but attainable, so you can build up confidence as you start reaching your goals. It's a fine balance, but using this mnemonic will get you on the right track.

Start by making a goal statement.

What would you like to achieve?

Write it down in the **S.M.A.R.T.** format, and keep it in a place you will see every day.

Revisit and readjust the statement if you have to, but try it out first. Put in some good, solid effort toward reaching it. After all, a goal without a plan is just a wish.

If you prefer to form your goal statements using an app instead, try **Lifetick**. This app helps you create **S.M.A.R.T.** goals, has a cheering squad, and also leaves you comments with extra motivation to help you reach your goals.

THE QUARTERLY PLAN

I have a client that hired me to get her in shape enough to walk two or three miles at a time so she can live her dream to travel the world and take photos. She is newly retired, but has been madly in love with Couch for the past year. She has gained 50lbs, developed a bad self-image, and feels plain rotten (Couch will do that to us, so beware). When we first met, she was anxious about starting an exercise program and learning to eat clean again. What seemed to be such a big task made her worry. We set her three-month goal to walk her neighborhood loop in ten minutes. At first, she could not even walk down the street without getting so winded and wobbly she had to turn around and head back home. We continued to exercise a few times each week to build up her endurance and functional strength. We set the goal for six months to walk the loop in under ten minutes. At the nine-month mark, we would walk the loop and down the road to another loop and back. By one year, she had booked for her own adventure to take photos at a farm in Vermont, which required many hours of walking over the course of a few days. By setting these goals each quarter, my client was able to stay on task, focus on her dreams, and make them a reality.

Goals give you something to aim for. Similar to having a scheduled vacation, setting goals gives you something to look forward to; however, it can be challenging to define and narrow down your aspirations. One thing I like my clients to do is to list short-term and long-term goals. A **SHORT-TERM GOAL** is one you want to reach in the first three months, and a **LONG-TERM GOAL** is what you want to accomplish one year from now. Time frames help you to focus on what's important now (that instant gratification we all crave) and what you want later (our future dreams). Doing this allows you to make realistic gains without getting sidetracked on your way.

Find something to reach for every quarter this year and create a goal sheet. It can be anything that dials you in on making some healthy changes, but plan for three, six, nine, and twelve months.

☐ Make the first goal (zero-three months) simple and the last goal (one year from now) challenging, yet attainable if you stay the course.

☐ Mark those end dates on your calendar.

Planning those quarter goals will help get your started and give you a real purpose for doing what you are doing.

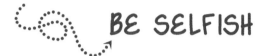

BE SELFISH

It's about you this time. You need to explore and discover your **W.I.IF M.** **W.I.IF M.** stands for *"What's In It for Me?"* The idea is that we all selfishly do things that provide some value to ourselves. It defines where your motivation comes from. For example, what do I get if I leave Couch? Perhaps more energy, followed by a slew of awesome choices? Since we are all naturally self-centered (even though we may try hard not to be), we want to get something out of the effort we have exerted. Answering **W.I.IF M.** helps narrow your focus down to two approaches for evaluating motivation: intrinsic and extrinsic motivation.

Intrinsic (or internal) motivation is that which comes from within. It is what would make you think of exercise with a smile. You embrace the opportunity to move more because you like how it makes you feel and know it will get you to your goal. You engage in exercise for pleasure.

Extrinsic motivation comes from external forces. For example, your spouse wants you to lose a few pounds, so he or she hires you a personal trainer; alternatively, perhaps you signed up for an exercise class at the gym just to get the free water bottle and t-shirt. Many people use some amount of extrinsic motivation for exercise. This would be engaging in exercise more for the known benefits, over the actual enjoyment of it. There are many influences that factor into the motivation story. What you have to decide is…what are yours?

I want you to make a list of both the intrinsic and extrinsic factors that may influence your exercise. They should be statements or reasons why you do or why you would exercise. Such as, *"I want to start exercising because…"* or *"I desire to be healthier because…"* Step back, and look at your list. Which statements make you feel good? Which statements have a negative connotation? Are you finding that you are exercising or starting to exercise for the right reasons? Focus on one reason that makes you the happiest, and put a big circle around it, highlight it, paste it on your wall…whatever works for you. Make sure to revisit your statement, and see if it really is a true motivator for you.

CHAPTER 8

SUMMARY

- You have to set goals if you want to be successful with your exercise plan along with many other aspects of your life.

- Create goals that are specific, measurable, attainable, realistic, and timely. These are also known as S.M.A.R.T. goals.

- Set both short-term and long-term goals. These help you plan for your present and future success. You never want to stop reaching for the stars.

- Determine your intrinsic and extrinsic motivation. Be selfish, and make it all about YOU this time!

CHAPTER 9

Get Picture Perfect

*"I dream, I test my dreams against my
beliefs, I dare to take risks, and I execute my
vision to make those dreams come true."*
—*Walt Disney*

What does your ideal date look like? All of us have a mental list of what we are looking for in a companion. We can picture them in our mind's eye. You must do the same when picturing your life without Couch. The key to creating a life filled with more activity and exercise is leaving Couch behind and out of sight. Get out as often as you can to search for your new love. Get out there, and move on.

Visual cues can make or break your success in reaching your exercise goals. You may have encountered this in other areas of your life. For instance, I usually put the vitamins on the kitchen counter, and my teenage son will come into the kitchen and take his vitamin. One day, I cleared off the counters for a fresh and clean look; without thinking, I put the vitamins in the cabinet. As a result, I noticed that my son did not take his vitamin for the next few days. Why? Out of sight out, of mind. Without a VISUAL REMINDER, he would forget to take his vitamins; but when the vitamins were on the counter, he would remember to take them. Do you get where I am going with this one? Ring! Ring! This is your wake-up call. The same goes for Couch.

A visual cue or trigger is a signal that reminds us to do something. The vitamin example can serve as example for getting workouts in. If your running pants are neatly tucked in a drawer, there is no visual cue to remind you. Use visuals as your tools. When you need a little motivation, items such as gym clothes, sneakers, and workout gear can be your saving grace. If your clothes and sneakers are laid out next to your bed, they will be staring you in the face in the morning. It will be much easier if there is no guessing, no other work for your brain, besides, having to put on your clothes and go! Be sure to place your gym items where you can see them. If you don't yet own any exercise gear, sneakers, or workout clothes, purchase enough for five days a week. Make your exercise a *"visual thing,"* and there will be no escape, no excuses, and no reason you won't succeed at getting your sweat on.

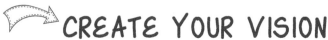 CREATE YOUR VISION

Making your dreams and goals visible creates belief. Visualization also makes you reflect on the question, *"What is*

it that I really want in life, and how can I make that happen?"
One tool I like to use with my clients is a vision board. Everyone
has their own style, so this can be a really fun and motivating
activity. I will outline what I have my clients do and you can try
it out yourself.

HOW TO CREATE
A VISION BOARD

» STEP 1: Decide what you would like to use as your "poster."
It can be a poster board, but there are no limits. Size depends
on where you decide to display it.

» STEP 2: Find a photo of yourself when you remember being
the happiest. The picture has nothing to do with age or weight.
It is more internal: you felt great, you were happy with who you
were as a person, and you had a good self-image. Think of why
you were this way. What were you doing then that you aren't
doing now? Place that photo in the middle, and surround it by
the remaining steps.

» STEP 3: Write down or put into print your **S.M.A.R.T.**
goal.

» STEP 4: Find a quote that inspires you.

» STEP 5: Develop a mantra. This is a statement you will say
when you are feeling weak or want to quit. It can be something
simple like, *"You got this"* or *"Just one more rep."*

» STEP 6: Place photos of what you want to achieve so you
have a visual. If you want to exercise so you can be healthy

enough to run after your grandkids, maybe add some pics of your grandkids. Make it personal, and have it show emotion with words such as *"Ahhh!"* or *"Yay!"*

>> STEP 7: If you have limited space or want to take your visions with you on your travels, try using Vision Board apps such as **iWish** or **Happy Tapper**. Commit to your vision and use awesome services created by the marvelous Janet Tanguay at www.hammockwayoflife.com. Here you can receive your own vision board in the mail, attend workshops, or work with a coach to make your dreams come true.

ENVISION A NEW LIFE

Mental imagery is a term used to describe what we visualize in the mind's eye, so to speak. You can think of it as fantasizing, dreaming, or imagining. World-class athletes do this. Some studies show that when athletes mentally visualize success, they have physical gains without physically training harder. For instance, an article from the *Journal of Sport & Exercise Psychology* (1996) proved that weightlifting imagery produced actual changes in the muscles. Having visualized the changes, athletes could imagine, feel, believe, and achieve better results. Isn't it crazy what our minds and bodies are capable of?

Another great example of this would be stated by the professional golfer, Jack Nicklaus. Nicklaus has won eighteen professional championships—the most any player has won in his career. He describes how he imagines every shot in his book, *Golf My Way*. He writes:

"I never hit a shot even in practice without having a sharp, in-focus picture in my head. It's like the color movie. First, I 'see' the ball where I want to finish, nice and white and sitting up high on the green grass. Then the scene quickly changes and I 'see' the ball going there; it's path, trajectory, shape, and even its behavior on landing. Then there's a sort of a fade out, and the next scene shows me making the kind of swing that will turn the previous images into reality. Only at the end of this short, private, Hollywood spectacular do I select a club and step up to the ball."

Envision your success with exercising. This will take some mental practice and mental dress rehearsals. Here are some simple ways to start with a daily daydream:

☐ Commit to five minutes at first, and set a timer.

☐ Go to a quiet space ,and close your eyes.

☐ Start to imagine yourself reaching your most-desired goal. For example, you want to be able to ride your bike for 30 minutes without having to stop and rest.

☐ Imagine you have already accomplished it. What does this feel like? Picture the details, even down to the socks you are wearing. By doing this, you will build your self-confidence and self-belief.

- ☐ Feel the emotion that goes along with reaching your goals. Practice receiving compliments from others, and feel what it would feel like to be in that moment. Are you excited, relieved, proud of yourself? Bask in your moment of glory, and linger on the feeling.

- ☐ Now, switch perspective. Pretend you are an outsider looking in. You are clapping and proud of that person who just reached their goal and are inspired to do so yourself.

- ☐ Gently open your eyes when the timer goes off. Make your next move an active one. Take the steps necessary to achieve your goal, and remember that feeling of being unstoppable.

Try to incorporate this into your daily routine. The more you envision yourself exercising, the more you will want to become your vision.

A PHOTO FINISH

Sometimes our minds play tricks on us. We think we look frumpy or have bigger saddle bags than we actually do. A visual of this is important to many people. Plus, we want to feel good about ourselves after all the positive changes we made through this breakup. There is a video clip on YouTube of a man who took a picture of his body for 365 days to show every detail of his progress. It's neat to watch how his body transforms through his year of exercise. It is why most success stories in those magazines provide a before and after picture of the person. It makes you step back and say, *"Wow."* Even if you take the picture and tuck it away in a shoebox in the far reaches of your closet, take it. You will be happy you did.

Here's how to take your transformation photos:

- ☐ Stand in front of your mirror wearing a bathing suit or tight-fitting clothes. Face the mirror with arms at your sides and feet together.

- ☐ Take a picture with your phone or camera.

- ☐ Turn to the side with your arms comfortably at your sides and take a profile picture.

- ☐ Now face the mirror and have someone take the picture of you from behind. You can also do this if you have a tripod, selfie stick, or a self-timing device.

- ☐ Save your photos in a safe place, and visit them when you feel you are making progress with your body shape.

- ☐ Take your "after" photos about every 6 weeks to track your progress. Use the same clothes, same time of day, same background, and same body position to keep things consistent.

CHAPTER 9

SUMMARY

- ✓ Make your active lifestyle a visual thing.

- ✓ Create a vision board to display your inspirational quotes, pictures, and goals.

- ✓ Use mental imagery to help you focus on who you really want to be.

- ✓ Take "before and after" photos to provide visuals on how your body is transforming. This provides a ton of motivation.

CHAPTER 10

Showing Signs of Progress

"Do not confuse motion with progress. A rocking horse keeps moving but does not make any progress."
—Alfred A. Montapert

She is on a roll. She starts strong by getting up early and working out at the local gym for twenty minutes every morning. Couch is begging for her to come back. Three weeks into it she hits the snooze button and misses a few workouts. Week four, no more early bird. She fizzles out and is back at Couch's comfy side by week five. Sound familiar?

I bet she did not track her progress. Maybe she wanted to see results *"like yesterday,"* so she ended that gym relationship. It's hard to push yourself if there is no record of what you have accomplished. Success stories are measured by results, specifically measureable results: *"I lost ten pounds; I lost two inches in my waist; I can do ten push-ups; I am walking ten thousand steps a day."*

Tracking your progress or daily activity can be a huge motivator. It not only shows you the concrete data, but again, provides you with a visual, a number, some form of solid evidence you have been looking for. Think of it as your medicine. You go to the doctor, she tells you that you have high blood pressure (measureable), to take blood pressure medication, and come back in four weeks. What does she do after four weeks? She measures your blood pressure, of course, to see if it you have made progress. Tracking your progress is another way to make your journey all the more "real." I warn you that if you do not go through these ho-hum motions, you will not see the changes. Instead, you will be frustrated that you are putting in time and getting nothing for it. As Valanetino Crawford said, *"You cannot change what you don't manage; you cannot manage what you don't track."*

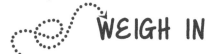

WEIGH IN

Yes, I am talking about getting on that scale. Weight is used to help figure out waist-to-hip ratios and BMIs, which certainly tell us important things about our health. Scales, however, are tools and only one piece of the healthy puzzle. I agree that weight is a very useful measurement for many reasons, but be careful! It can cripple you if you become too obsessed with it.

I am here to tell you that weight does not come *on* overnight, therefore it will not come *off* overnight. If you know you gained 20lbs this year, then it's not the dinner you had last night or the party you hosted this weekend that packed those pounds on.

The weight is a collection of the dinners, parties, and decisions you have made over the past year. It is an increase that has built up over time due to eating more calories than you are burning. Are you compounding the calories or creating a calorie deficit?

If your goal is to lose weight or gain weight, weigh yourself once a week. When you see that your weight each week continues to go in the direction you want consistently, then what you are doing is working. Another thing to note is that you should have a physical and bloodwork done every year. Thyroid malfunctions, low iron levels, new medications, hormonal imbalances, certain diseases, syndromes, and many other factors can affect your weight, so make sure you are getting the best out of your exercise by getting your health taken care of first.

Here is my advice about the scale: Weigh yourself on the day you decide to start your fitness journey. Do this first thing in the morning with no clothes on, before you eat, and after you use the bathroom. Record this number in your journal. Then follow my golden rule: weigh yourself once a week on the same day in the same way. Do this for 6 weeks. If after this period the number on the scale upsets you, lose it (the scale, that is). If it motivates you, use it. Do what will cause you the least amount of stress, and focus instead on the way you feel, not necessarily the number on the scale. It's good to know your number, but do not to let it define you. Try out the **Happy** **Scale** app if you are searching for a simple weight loss tracker that will show you your very own weight loss trends. Set your own goals, and even get motivational photos.

MEASURE IT

Measurements show a bigger picture. You can gain muscle and lose inches but still not budge the scale. Taking measurements is a great method for tracking how your body shape is changing as you get more fit. It is a huge motivator! Where you hold your weight matters as well. Apple shapes are more at risk for disease than pear shapes. Waist-to-hip ratios are used for this reason.

Take your measurements on the day you decide to start your fitness journey. First, purchase an inexpensive fabric tape measure (one that does not stretch). Second, make sure you are wearing tight fitting clothes or none at all (oh, yeah!) to decrease margins of error. Lastly, start from the neck, and continue down to your calves. Make sure you measure before your workout, so there is no muscle pump or sweat affecting the results. Take your measurements at least twice to make sure they are the correct and consistent.

>> NECK: Measure across the Adam's apple.

>> CHEST: Measure directly across your nipple line.

>> WAIST: Measure the narrowest point width-wise.

>> WAIST-BELLY BUTTON: Measure at the belly button.

>> WAIST-WIDEST: Measure the widest part (this is not always at the belly button, so that is why I do all three waist measurements).

>> **HIPS:** With feet together, measure the widest part of the hip-bones and across the widest part of the buttocks.

>> **THIGH:** Measure around the fullest part (measure about ten inches up from the top of the knee cap for standardization).

>> **CALVES:** Measure the thickest part (measure from the bottom of the knee cap down, so you can measure the same spot next time).

>> **BICEP:** Measure at maximum circumference with arms extended, relaxed, and with palms facing forward. You can also flex your muscle and measure that, too!

>> **FOREARMS:** Measure from the elbow (about five inches down for standardization purposes).

reminder

Have the same person take your measurements for consistency purposes.

SHOP IN YOUR CLOSET

This is a combo platter of weight and measurements without even knowing it. If you have no scale and no measuring tape, just visit your closet. Some of my clients have the goal to "*be able to fit into my skinny jeans again*." It is not a bad goal, as long as your skinny jeans aren't from the sixth grade. Be realistic here. If those skinny jeans were from a few years ago, it's realistic. Feeling good in your skin (or in this case, your skinny jeans) is sometimes more important than weight and measurement. After all, you're getting back into the dating game, so you have to look and feel your best. You know if you can get into those jeans (without using lard rubbed all over your legs and needing two of your friends to help you button them up) then you will feel like you have achieved your goal. It's important to track how your clothes are fitting and reflect on when you feel your best. What are you wearing? How do those clothes and the way they fit your body make you feel? Confidence is sexy all the way around.

On the other side of the coin, get rid of your "chubby clothes." We all have had that stash of clothes or a few items that we dedicate to our plumper size. When you reach your goal and get back into those "next-size-down" jeans, donate the bigger clothes. **DO NOT** save them "just in case." This gives yourself permission to go back and gain some weight later on. You have worked hard for those skinny jeans, so toss the frumpy ones. I don't care how comfortable they are. Be confident: you like the way you are and you are not going back to the size that made you unhappy and unhealthy. You would be setting yourself up for failure. If you gain the weight back, you will have to feel the pain of buying a whole new wardrobe. This might be enough motivation to keep you on track. Here is your assignment:

☐ Be a closet shopper and find one outfit that is way too big and frumpy that you can donate. Put it in a bag and drop it off at your local donation drop-off.

☐ Take out that favorite pair of pants or top that is a size too small and use it as your motivation.

☐ If you don't have any clothes that are a size too small, buy some!

☐ Put your "goal clothes" up front and center in your closet, where you can see them every day. If you build it, they will come!

A LITTLE SOMETHING EXTRA

It's important to measure your gains in other ways besides the size and shape of your body. There are many posture and movement assessments used to measure physical capabilities. I will not overcomplicate it, but instead provide you with a few simple forms of assessment I use with my clients. You should pick a few to complete every three months. If in doubt, hire a professional to help you. Many personal trainers will meet with you for a consult and test all of these (and more) for you if you ask.

>> **VO2max:** VO2max measures your efficiency to take in oxygen at maximal exertion. It is measured to provide you with information about your overall condition and cardiorespiratory efficiency. You can get fancy and hooked up to specialized equipment in a lab, or you can find an estimate by testing it in your very own home (or have a professional help you with it.)

>> **SIT AND REACH:** The sit and reach test is used to measure how flexible you are, particularly in your hamstrings and lower back muscles. This test is very general, but it is important since tightness in these areas can be the root of back pain (which is all too common in our society).

>> **HEEL TO TOE WALK:** Walk the imaginary tight rope, baby! This simple test is used to assess balance. This exercise may seem easier than it actually is. Balance is needed throughout all stages in life, not only to prevent injury, but also because balance is a component of all movement.

>> **OVERHEAD SQUAT:** This is used to assess dynamic flexibility on both sides of the body, as well as total body strength. It is meant to identify weak and strong muscles and movement compensations.

>> **THE PLANK:** This isometric move is the true test of core strength by doing nothing other than holding still. Basic but challenging, hold and time yourself with perfect form.

CHAPTER 10

SUMMARY

- ✅ Use the scale as a tool to track your progress for six to twelve weeks.

- ✅ Take your measurements to find your waist-to-hip ratio. This will help you assess the changes in the shape of your body by using concrete numbers.

- ✅ Get rid of your old clothes and find the ones that will build your confidence. Use a smaller size for motivation.

- ✅ Track your flexibility, balance, cardio efficiency, and strength, depending on your goal.

CHAPTER 11

Get All Decked Out

"You can have anything you want in life
if you dress for it."

—*Edith Head*

You want to look your finest when approaching the "dating" world. If you are going to be serious about your health and fitness, you have to look the part. The good news is that there are many wearable accessories that can provide you with the motivation and accountability you need to get his done.

The "tech" part of fitness can help all kinds of people get started on their journey to a more active lifestyle. Take Jimmy, for instance. He had absolutely no interest in working out. Jimmy was a big fan of technology—and that required a ton of sitting. His job consisted of programming software, fixing computers, and purchasing whatever new device Apple had to offer. His relationship with tech led to years of unwanted weight gain. When I first met Jimmy, he was turned off by exercise of any kind. He was not a "gym guy," as he put it, and had no desire to change. His doctor, however, broke the news that he had a fatty liver that would get worse unless he lost some significant weight. That's when Jimmy reached out to me. I knew during his first session that we had to incorporate his passion into his exercise program. We played some games on the X-box Kinect that required us to stand, jump, dodge, and run. Jimmy also decided to get a Fitbit that tracked his daily steps and activity. He loved the reports it would give him and the syncability with his phone. The blend of "tech" and fitness was what it took to get—and keep—him moving.

Activity trackers, heart rate monitors, pedometers, and other exercise-tracking gizmos are the new must-have accessories. They are also great devices to keep you on track and measure your progress, as I discussed in the last chapter. Some devices measure a multitude of factors, but the question of which one you should pick depends upon your goals and what you are trying to achieve by wearing the device. Some people love to play with things and these tech "toys" can get and keep them motivated. If you are one of those people, read on. This may be what you need.

TAKE ACTION STEPS

A pedometer is a wearable device used to track your steps. You can wear them in multiple ways, depending on your preference. Tracking your steps every day is a great way to gauge how much you move. If you are looking to maintain your weight, 10,000 steps per day is the recommendation. If you are looking to lose weight, 12,000-14,000 steps daily is better! These wearables also offer tracking for activity, sleep, calories, and more. Here are some of the leading products and my favorite picks (based on my own experience and feedback from clients and friends). Also note that these companies have products that can be clipped on instead of being worn around the wrist. I am also aware that these will be forever changing as the technology evolves. If you are partial to Samsung or Apple- they have watches available as well that sync to your phone and all of that fancy stuff!

Fitbit Charge: This device tracks sleep, steps, calories, and even displays incoming calls! This slick wrist band is water resistant but not waterproof.

The Jawbone Up24: This wearable tracks sleep and steps. The app is awesome; it provides great graphs, allows you to input personalized goals, and reminds you to get up and move around. There is no touch screen on this tracker, but it is light, stylish, and easy to wear.

Garmin Vivofit: The screen shows basic sleep tracking, steps, calories burned, and reminders to get up and move. This band does not need to be plugged in because the battery is rated to last one full year.

MisFit Flash: The device not only tracks sleep, steps, distance, and calories, but it is also completely waterproof and can be worn while swimming for all those aqua divas out there! The coin battery lasts six months and is easy to replace. The tracker can be worn on your wrist or waist with an included clip-on accessory.

🕐 **MisFit Shine:** This band is stylish and comes with fancy accessories. Where this one shines is with its sleep-tracking ability. It knows when you are asleep without you having to push any buttons. It gives you every detail of your sleep pattern down to deep-sleep, light-sleep, and even REM patterns.

FIND YOUR HEART THROB

These contraptions track your heart rate and physical exertion. By allowing you to know your real-time heart rate information, these devices help you to stay on pace, work harder, or know when to back it down. There are plenty to choose from, so depending on your budget and what you want in a tracker, you can have your pick. Heart rate monitors typically consist of a wrist-watch display and a chest strap containing an electrode. The technology has become more advanced, however, so some monitors do not require the chest strap. Just do your research and check out the product reviews before you purchase one (and don't worry, these monitors come with directions to help you figure out what your heart rate should be). Here are my favorite wearables that include heart rate monitors:

🕐 **Fitbit Charge HR:** An activity tracker and heart rate monitor. It uses continuous heart rate and constant, accurate feedback. The touch screen shows daily stats. No chest strap necessary for this one, and you still get your sleep, steps, and calorie information (I currently use it and LOVE it).

Basis Peak: This watch provides continuous heart rate monitoring and is known for being very simple to use and extremely accurate. It can auto-detect when you are running and will provide you all of your stats on a web app. No chest strap required.

Polar FT4: This tracker is the size of an average watch and will not only track heart rate, but it will also tell you what heart rate zones you should be in for your best workout. It also keeps track of your previous workouts. It is simple for beginners to set up and use and it requires the use of a chest strap.

Mio Alpha: This sports watch does not require a chest strap, allowing for continuous heart rate monitoring. It calculates calories burned and can also be used with your smartphone GPS.

ACCESSORIZE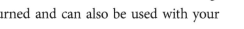

There are some other fun and techy activity gadgets on the market that will motivate you to ditch Couch and accessorize your fitness. I am sure that by the time this book gets published, there will some new devices on the market. Welcome to the twenty-first century, everyone! For now, here are a few of my suggestions.

FOR RUNNERS AND CYCLISTS:

>> **GARMIN EDGE 800 CYCLE COMPUTER:** This device is a touchscreen minicomputer that has GPS navigation and built-in maps. It is meant to withstand bad weather, bumps, and knocks (yoohoo, mountain bike riders and trail runners). It also stores distance, speed, and elevation.

>> **SENSORIA SMART SOCK:** A running sock that gives your ankle feedback. It tracks how you have been running and how you can improve over time. There is a virtual coach to help. The socks are washable, thank goodness! www.sensoriafitness.com

FOR TAKING WEIGHT:

>> **Fitbit Aria Scale:** The scale comes with Wi-Fi. It not only takes your weight, but will measure your BMI, body fat percentage, and keeps track of your numbers.

FOR THE SPORTS JUNKIE:

>> **Go Pro Hero:** This action camera can attach to your chest or your helmet. It is waterproof and shock-proof. Take photos or video of yourself doing your most awesome stunts. We use this for our summer adventures on the boat. It makes cliff jumping a high, adrenaline experience for the whole family!

>> **Trace:** This activity tracker fits on to your surfboards, skateboards, and snowboards. It is shockproof, waterproof, and durable.

>> **Amiigo:** The tracker band goes around your wrist and feet. It can be used to track activity in cycling, swimming, walking, hiking, biking, water sports, weight-lifting, and cardio.

FOR THE SWIMMER:

>> **Finis Neptune:** This MP3 player can be used in the water. You secure this bone conduction device to your swim goggles. It allows you to listen to music without using earbuds. Super awesome!

INVEST IN A PAIR

Any fashion guru will tell you that "the shoes make the outfit." They are the staple that brings it all together. You have to not only look good, but also feel good when jumping into the exercise-dating world. Out of all the pieces of equipment you can invest in when starting to exercise, shoes are the most important. Support starts from the ground up. Not having the proper footwear can really hinder your progress and result in muscle imbalances that will ultimately lead to injury.

Connie was having hip and knee pain every time she walked for an extended period of time. Her chiropractor, massage therapist, and physical therapist helped re-align her spine and worked on eradicating muscle pains on a weekly basis. It wasn't until she decided to see an orthopedic specialist that she learned that she needed inserts and custom supportive shoes. Connie's orthopedist was not happy to hear that she had been walking in sandals! When she started to wear her new inserts and shoes around the house and during errands, she noticed a difference. At first, her muscles were sore but in different areas then before. Within a week, she could walk pain-free. Many clients of mine, similar to Connie, notice differences in joint pain when they switch shoes or are not wearing adequate footwear. The basic rule is to invest in new footwear every three hundred miles or six months (whichever comes first). When was the last time you invested in some new kicks? If your new shoes are still not giving you enough support, it may be worth making an appointment with a specialist like a podiatrist.

There are shoes for every type of exercise. Make sure to get supportive footwear based on your goals. For example, if your goal is to hike, get some good hiking boots. If you are getting into cross training and weightlifting, don't limit yourself to running sneakers. Shoes all serve a purpose in different ways. Don't just purchase some because they look spiffy (though that is always a plus). If you are going to spend a decent amount of money, they should be functional too. Visit a reputable specialty store, and speak with the experts. Here is what you should know about your feet before you visit the store to do some shopping:

☐ Do you have flat feet, a high arch, or a neutral foot? If you don't know, check out *"How to Use the Footprint"* test on **www.wikihow.com** and try it out.

☐ Is one foot bigger than the other?

☐ Have someone take pictures of your stride, running or walking. Do you run/walk on your heels, mid-foot? Do your feet pronate or supinate?

☐ Tell the sales person what type of activity you are going to be doing in your shoes. Be specific. Some stores may even have you walk/jog around so they can take a gait analysis.

☐ Purchase more than one pair of shoes for each activity, if you need to. I have fifteen pairs—all for different activities. It can be expensive but your body will thank you. Plus, you'll always look stylish!

CHAPTER 11

SUMMARY

- Invest in an activity tracker or pedometer to track your progress.

- If you are trying to improve on your cardio fitness, try using a heart rate monitor to measure your heart rate and level of exertion.

- Check out the other gizmos on the market if you are a tech-junkie. There is one for every kind of activity.

- Pick the right shoe for your activity. You don't want to increase your chances of injury—and you need the best support you can get.

CHAPTER 12

Visit the Dating Scene

"If you want to be seen, you have to put yourself out there- it's that simple."
—Karin Fossum

You're getting over your neediness for Couch and are moving on. Why not tell surrounding nations? We live in a world that is now inundated with streams of social media and networking platforms. New programs are developed every day. Some people enjoy being able to speak freely and take a stand when they can write it, post it, pin it, tweet it, hashtag it, poke it, and whatever else there is now. They are great tools for getting back out into the exercise-dating scene. Let the world know about the new you and what you are looking for.

Psychologists and researchers alike have studied the effects of social media and posting public statements or claims about your health. The consensus is that letting everyone know what you are doing helps you stay loyal to your choices. Some weight-loss clinics force their clients to write down and show their weight-loss goal to their friends, relatives, and neighbors. These clinics have discovered that this works when other things have failed. It requires more work than just telling a friend— and there is cold, hard, evidence in black and white. As Ray F. Baumeister puts it, *"A failure, a slip-up, a lapse in self-control can be swept under the carpet pretty easily if you are the only one who knows about it."* Putting your results out there allows you to take the burden off of monitoring yourself because now everyone else can do it for you. Others can also motivate you by cheering you on for sticking with it and doing such a great job. Who doesn't want that pat on the back? Public commitments can produce a change within, and it may be just what you need to help you reach your goals, no matter how big or how small.

→ TELL THE WORLD

Think of your Facebook buddies who have posted something about starting their journey with weight loss, diet, or exercise. Not only do we like it when friends support us and cheer us on, but their encouragement also helps to keep us accountable. If you usually post your sweaty face after each workout, but you don't feel like going to the gym today…missing a sweaty selfie post may be enough to motivate you to go. As Robert Cialdini writes in his national bestseller, *"Whenever someone takes a stand that is visible to others, there arises a drive to maintain that stand in order to look like a consistent person"* (from *Influence: the Psychology of Persuasion*). In other words, people don't want to look uncertain, fickle, scatterbrained, or unstable. The drive to be and look consistent, Robert suggests, constitutes a highly-potent weapon of social influence. Using social platforms like Facebook, Instagram, Twitter, and even LinkedIn can be powerful tools to propel you forward and help you reach your goals.

Social media is also an avenue where people get ongoing support without limits. If you think about it, your contacts are not only your best buds, but they also include people from work, acquaintances, family members, even people you hardly know. Evidence shows that positive support can keep you motivated and this is what you get with social media. Researchers at the University of South Carolina's Arnold School of Public Health found participants who regularly tweeted status updates such as, *"I avoided eating a pastry this morning at a breakfast meeting,"* lost more weight. Tracking devices mentioned in the last section, such as Fitbit and Jawbone, also have social aspects. You can make your profile public so that your network can see everything you are doing. This may sound creepy to some, but it really works!

BE A PART OF THE COMMUNITY

It is difficult to stay loyal to your goals when you feel isolated or separated from your community. Take Karen, for instance. Karen reached out to me desperate for help; over the phone, she began to tell me that although she wanted so badly to continue to lead an active life, she was bound to her wheelchair most of the day. She explained that because she had little family living in the area, she had nobody to assist her with driving to the pool, gym, or anywhere else in general. Since her condition confined her to living in senior housing (even though she is in her 50s), Karen was struggling to find services to help her get around (as those services tended to be reserved for seniors only.) Even when I recommended a traveling physical therapist to her, she felt that it helped but just *"not enough."* She felt alone and helpless. Without a supportive community, Karen felt (and really was) trapped.

As Karen explained to me, working out (or living) without a community is like going through the motions but without any real sense of accomplishment. It was not until I recommended a company called Community Connection to her that she felt liberated. With the introduction of this group of volunteers, Karen had a support system that would drive her to her appointments, cook for her, take her out on errands, and sometimes just come and visit. Karen reached out me to tell me about how wonderful the program was—and about how they were even taking her to the pool now! In Karen's words, *"This all has a benefit to me and I'm not feeling so isolated."* The eye-opener for us here is that you never know what's out there until you put some effort in to find it.

A great example of community that comes to my mind when I think of a fitness world would be CrossFit. CrossFit incorporates a mix of aerobic, gymnastics, and Olympic weight lifting exercises. These gyms are known for being *"intense"* and provide many levels of fitness competition. Some tout these groups as *"crazy"*, *"to the extreme"*, or even *"cultish."* Though I have done some CrossFit training/exercises on my own, I have never trained in a CrossFit gym. I know that my many CrossFit pals out there absolutely love it and not just because they feel totally badass: they love it because of the support and sense of community they get in and out of the gym environment. Everyone there is aiming for the same goal—they all want to push themselves and see the results of their hard work. When you have those similarities and people all around you that are supportive, you become successful at achieving your goals. I know CrossFit is not for everyone but it's one example of the community we all seem to be searching for.

The mere satisfaction of gaining support from others does not have to start in the gym environment. It can be in the community in which you reside. When your community begins to provide support and assistance to your friends and neighbors, it helps to build that bond of community itself. With your community, you will find new, great ways to socialize, exercise, and raise money for causes you are passionate about. Here are a few ideas for checking out what your local community has to offer:

□ Grab a Penny Saver or your free community paper to take a look in the health and wellness section.

□ Health Fairs are perfect for finding information, getting free samples, listening to the experts, and trying out some fitness classes.

□ Attend an open house at a local health club. Often, there are free classes and a chance to talk to experts.

□ Participate in a park clean-up day.

□ Help a neighbor with yard work.

□ Attend an active fundraiser or church function.

□ Participate in a community walk or sign up to be one of the volunteers to cheer those walkers on!

□ **www.Meetup.com** is a great site for finding locals that want to get together to share something, learn something, or do something together.

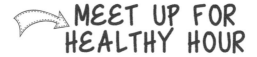

MEET UP FOR HEALTHY HOUR

When scientists studied eighty year olds, they found that those who were the most social suffered seventy percent less cognitive decline than the least social bunch. It gives us all the more reason to be social. There are some new clubs (mostly in the major cities like Boston, New York, Chicago, and LA) that offer a healthy hour as opposed to happy hour. You get together for an hour and exercise, and then stay to eat some food and drink protein shakes. Some clubs even offer organic beer and wine after your workout. Natalie Bushaw, a spokeswoman for Life Time Fitness, says that people who *"sweat to be social"* love it because they have accomplished two things: catching up and working out. Penny Love Hoff, Head of Life Time Athletic in Harrison, New York started a 45-minute barre class (ballet and other exercises while holding onto stationary handrail for support) followed by a 15-minute bar. Participants stick to the schedule and are always on time!

If you are from a small town like I am, those clubs may be hard to find. Hint...this is an untapped market out there! An easier way to incorporate this idea would be to try a night out doing something active. Instead of happy hour, try going to do something that requires being active and social. Instead of having a weekly meeting at the bar with your pals, try meeting up to do something active. If you feel you need a drink in your hand, try a fresh fruit smoothie. The possibilities for those are endless! You may be surprised that your old happy hour at the bar or plopped on the couch after a long day just isn't cutting it anymore. You may find that your new hour of breaking a sweat makes you a happier, healthier person. Couch is at home lounging away while you are out finding a new love with your pals.

Don't forget to try a night out doing something active.

Here are a few *happy hour* ideas to help you get started:

- ☐ Walk around town for an hour and enjoy the sites.
- ☐ Find a nice bike path and ride your bike to dinner.
- ☐ Play a round of golf after work.
- ☐ Take a yoga class to de-stress from your day.
- ☐ Try indoor rock-climbing. Don't knock it until you try it.
- ☐ Go for a trail run/jog/walk with a group of pals.
- ☐ Find and attend a Happy Hour fitness party if there are gyms in your town or city that offer these types of classes. You don't know unless you ask around or search for these classes in your area.

CHAPTER 12

SUMMARY

- Use social media to keep you accountable and get the support you need to keep going.

- Get involved in community events and causes that will keep you active and connect you with others that have the same goal.

- Make your happy hour, your active hour.

CHAPTER 13

Keeping Things Exciting

"Change is hard at first, messy in the middle, and gorgeous at the end."
—*Robin Sharma*

You have to keep things exciting if you want a new relationship to last. Now that you have been "dating" and finding new interests, you may find you need to spice things up a bit every now and then, so this new relationship with exercise doesn't get stale. If you are doing the same things, you will see the same results. If you don't change something, then nothing will ever change. If it does not challenge you, it does not change you. Nothing ever worth doing is easy…and so on, and so forth. You have heard these statements before, but what are you doing about them? Are you taking action or becoming stale, just like that peanut butter and jelly sandwich you've been making for lunch every day since you were seven years old?

I believe a lack of motivation can be narrowed down to one simple concept…the inability to change. Maybe you are not motivated to exercise because it bores you to tears. Perhaps you are frustrated because even though you have been going to the gym every day for over a year now, you are still not seeing the results you want. Maybe you are depressed and would rather cry to Couch and wallow in self-pity all day. Chances are, the problem stems from not breaking out of your tiny comfort zone. Changing this alone could get you to the very top of the success mountain without even getting out of breath!

In *Who Moved My Cheese?*, Spencer Johnson tells the tale of four characters who desperately search for cheese. A fast and simple read, this story's message is crystal clear: *"Be Ready To Change Quickly And Enjoy It Again & Again."* Change is a good thing and it is what allows us to grow and develop as human beings. Relationships (even with our exercise routines) need to change in order to maintain that spark—the butterflies-in-your-stomach kind of feeling. Apply these simple concepts to your exercise regimen, and watch as you burn with desire to be active.

CHANGE UP THE SCENERY

If you have switched up your exercises but still seem to be lacking gusto, try a new place to get your sweat on. Changing up the scenery can do wonders. It allows you to challenge your body in new ways and prevent you from plateau and boredom. I have a client who I meet in a new place for every workout. I am not saying you have to go to these extremes, but maybe the gym is just too drab. Take your workouts outdoors or head to a friend's house, join a new gym, start a neighborhood walking club, or try out a new trail each week. You have to switch things up to stay engaged and encourage muscular maintenance, growth, and endurance.

Experts like Eva Selhub, MD, co-author of *Your Brain on Nature,* report that exercising outdoors increases the likelihood that you will stick with a training program. How's that for motivation? If you enjoy it, you are more likely to do it again. Amen! Another advantage is the different terrain, which challenges your muscles differently than the flat environment of the gym. Outside, you will find elements like wind, rain, hills, and uneven turf. Because you don't know what to expect, things can be much more exciting. If you like walking but are bored of the treadmill or you are no longer seeing the results it used to give you, try walking outdoors. Switch up the places; add some hills or trails, or even change from walking on gravel to walking or running on sand in order to incorporate different muscles. To top it off, we know that spending time in nature has been linked to cognitive restoration. Getting out is like hitting the reset button on your stressed-out brain!

Exercising outdoors increases the likelihood that you will stick to a training program.

I challenge you to go on a fitness adventure. Try these suggestions to get started this week.

□ Exercise in a brand new place. How invigorating!

□ Discover what it is like to exercise in a totally different element, like sand, water, hills, woods, grass, etc.

□ Explore apps like Leafsnap (scan a photo of any leaf and the app will tell what kind of tree it is from), iBird Pro (ID different species of birds and play bird calls), or use RootsRated for outdoor ideas. All you have to do is enter your location and this app will give you an activity, directions, and some suggestions from local experts.

□ Take a fitness field trip. Bring the kids or ask friends for suggestions, and see if they want to accompany you.

KEEP 'EM GUESSING

Reaching a plateau can not only be frustrating but it can be so boring you would rather stick a few toothpicks in your eyes. Doing the same thing all of the time can be very stale and force you to lack bigtime in the motivation department. Muscle confusion is the concept that changing things up will force your muscles to transform and adapt. It's a good way to keep the body guessing. Here are a few simple ways to keep things fresh:

☐ Change up your cardio—Try a totally different machine from the "comfort-zone cardio" you are in. You can also add in inclines, intervals, or go backwards on some of the machines. By doing this, you will increase and challenge your cardio endurance. Have fun, get crazy.

☐ Find different exercises—Get a magazine or fitness book and find the exercises you have never done. Try them out. It will help you discover muscles you never knew you had, even those tiny muscles deep underneath!

☐ Change your grip: Switching your grip from overhand to underhand or narrow to wide can challenge your muscles in a new way. For example, when you complete an overhand grip pull up, you're primarily working your lats (the broadest muscle in your back) but when you change the grip to underhand during a pull-up, you are working your biceps (the major muscles in your upper arms). It's still a "pull-up" motion but you'll work a totally different muscle group. This goes to show you that small changes can yield completely different results.

☐ Add more sets—Try to add more sets than you typically do. One more set can bring you to the next level by building strength endurance to your major muscle groups.

☐ Complete more/fewer reps—Try more weight with less reps and less weight with more reps. More reps will incorporate long, lean, muscle, while fewer reps will help build strength and produce more "bulk."

☐ Try a new exercise modality—If you love lifting weights and have been doing it forever, try a new gig like Pilates, yoga, or dance. It challenges the body in a whole new way.

☐ Go slower or faster—If you do everything at the same speed, you need to change it up. For example, try lifting weights slower. It does not allow for the muscle to "get a break" and will increase muscle tone and endurance. You can also try running faster on the treadmill, instead of slow and steady. Small bursts of high intensity exercise are proven to torch some serious calories.

☐ Be still or jump—Try doing some isometric exercises (holding a position while your muscles are contracted like, yoga poses or the famous plank) or plyometrics (think box jumps and burpees). These are challenging for all levels of fitness from, beginners to conditioned athletes. Holding increases balance and strength in the stabilizer muscles, while jumping produces power and increased joint mobility.

☐ Use different equipment—There are so many pieces of equipment to choose from that challenge your muscles in a different way. Don't just stick to the same old thing. Try kettlebells, slides, medicine balls, BOSU balls, stability balls, resistance bands, bodyweight, dumbbells, barbells, cables, pulleys, sandbags, machines, boxes, suspension trainers…you get the point. There is a whole new world just waiting for you out there!

GOAL CHANGER

Joanne was not able to plank for more than five seconds when we started working together. By the end of six months, she could plank for over one minute. Go, Joanne! The next goal we set for her was to walk 10,000 steps daily, since she averaged about 6,000 steps per day. While doing so, along with some increased exercising, her knee was overwhelmed and started to bother her. We had to readjust her goal. Another exercise that was difficult for her was a V-sit. Same as the plank, what started off with five seconds turned into a minute. It made her ask the question. *"What next?"* Since she was more concerned about function and healthier living, we did not form goals around weight loss or losing inches. Her desires and focus changed from goals centered on her performance, to goals centered on eating clean foods rich in nutrients to not only strengthen her muscles, but to help her whittle her middle! Her goal was to cook one meal from her *Cooking Light* magazine each week and progresses from there. It would be new and different for her, but she was excited about the challenge and her newfound motivation.

Goals can't always stay the same. There is a difference between weight-loss goals, performance goals, and personal-growth goals. It's good to re-evaluate them on a consistent basis and switch things up. Reason being, if you have made a weight-loss goal and you have reached that goal, you may not be motivated to keep exercising. You need to discover the *"what's next?"* and create excitement to keep moving forward. Whatever your goals are, make sure you are constantly challenging yourself in different ways. Challenge yourself to do more and be more. If your goals are not changing, you're at a standstill—and that's pretty boring if you ask me.

CHAPTER 13

SUMMARY

- Change the scenery, and explore the outdoors!

- Use muscle confusion to keep transforming your body. Try new exercises, equipment, and modalities to create change.

- Evaluate your goals, and make sure you are changing them often.

PART 3

Having Fun

Enjoying Exercise, Your New Soul Mate

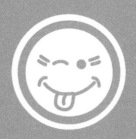

CHAPTER 14

Laugh Out Loud

"Find an exercise you love and you will never have to work out a day in your life."
—*Unknown*

Who doesn't love a good laugh? A laugh alone can make your new love more attractive and make you want to come back tomorrow night. I think I can say with 110% confidence that people want and need to have fun. It's right up there with oxygen and water!

We often postpone, delay, and avoid things we dread doing. Don't look at exercise this way. Find a form of exercise that you actually enjoy so you will be motivated to do it more often. It does wonders for those "feel good" emotions of ours. Exercise is known to be as effective as anti-depressant medication at relieving depression and boosting your mood. It can help you cope with life's challenges in a positive way. Happiness should not to be overlooked. I am not saying you should be laughing hysterically during your workouts (though with a good friend, this is a definite possibility). If you are working hard, you will be winded, red in the face, and unable to talk, let alone laugh. I get it. And there are times for these types of workouts. However, I do not think exercise should be looked at like a full-time job that we need to be serious, miserable, and overly tough about. It is important to find something enjoyable about your workout—something to look forward to and something that will make you feel downright happy. Even on the days I am stressed to the max, I try make my activity enjoyable in some way. It is good therapy for the soul. So grab a friend, take a long walk with your dog, try a yoga class in the park, or perhaps a Zumba dance party, and let's go have some fun!

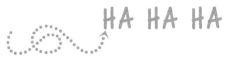

HA HA HA

Everyone laughs in the same language, and one of laughter's perks is that it is great exercise. Think of a friend of yours who has a contagious laugh. Their laugh makes you laugh. Or perhaps that guy in the crowd who bursts out laughing and it makes you giggle. There are wonderful benefits to laughing. As the saying goes, *"Laughter is the best medicine."* Some of those medicinal benefits include an increase in your heart rate, happiness, and test scores; the strengthening of bonds, your immune system, and pain tolerance; and a boost to your energy, your ability to release stress, and the amount of calories you burn. Laughing all day shouldn't be your only form of exercise, but it keeps you in a good mood, which may encourage you to hit your sweat session and officially make Couch your ex!

Loretta LaRoche, a stress-management consultant and the author of *Life is Short-Wear Your Party Pants* states, *"It's hard to laugh and be stressed at the same time."* Try it. Spin around in a circle and announce what is bothering you out loud. Feel better? I often make my clients do silly jacks (an exercise that works your oblique muscles, but makes you giggle because of how silly the movement looks) if they are having a low-energy kind of day. It gives us both a little chuckle and encourages a feel-good attitude. Here are a few ways to generate laughter when Couch is trying to lure you back in:

☐ Try laughter yoga. This class will help you get your laugh on! It is extremely fun and weird at the same time. The practice involves prolonged, voluntary laughter. To read more or to find an instructor in your area, go to laughteryoga.org You can also download their free laughing yoga guide, and try it out at home.

☐ Visit sites like Gigglers TV, a video channel dedicated to the funniest laughs online; College Humor, The Onion, and 9Gag.

☐ Check out Funniest Home Videos or Epic Fail compilations on YouTube, laughter is free, my friends!

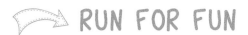 RUN FOR FUN

If you check out my website gallery, you will see the crazy outfits and runs I have done with some of my clients and good friends. I find that when people sign up for a race that is fun, they are more likely to try it, even if they have never walked a 5K, let alone run one. Some people run for the love of running, some people run to compete, and some people run for fun. If one of your goals is to run a 5K, I encourage you to sign up for a fun one. Plan an outfit and dress up with your friends, or register for a race that appeals to you. Anyone can do it. Bad knees, dislike cardio…doesn't matter. I want to let you in on a little secret…you don't have to run the whole time. Some people jog a little or walk when they need to. No one is watching you, and no one cares. You don't have to run because you love the act of running. You can run because you love the atmosphere of cheering crowds, the camaraderie, a challenge, a cool t-shirt, and a fun party afterwards. Just do it. It's not as bad as you think, but you have to experience it to know. There are runs in all sorts of weather and terrain, so find one that tickles your fancy. If you still need to ease into the racing scene, use some tools to make your "trying out this running thing" more enjoyable. Visit these websites for example, and explore some apps that may motivate you to get training, get running, and encourage you to have fun.

》Blood Sweat and Cheers (now part of Greatlist): Visit this site for beginner-friendly events that merge *"happy hour"* with your workout. This website has wonderful ideas, great articles, and fun events, and even cool fitness gear.

》Zombie's, Run!: It's a cross between a video game and an audiobook while you run. You complete missions, gather supplies, and come back to build up your village online. This app keeps you in suspense.

》Missile Wars: Avoid explosions while you run. Move solider!

》Charity Miles: This GPS-enabled app tracks mileage and raises money for all sorts of different causes. It's a great feeling to put in those miles for a cause you feel strongly about.

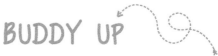

BUDDY UP

Friends don't let friends sit on the couch all day and melt away like slugs. True friends pull you up out of the couch cushions and force you to get out of your slump. Numerous studies prove that exercising with a partner or buddy helps motivate you and increases your intensity. A recent study from Stanford University found that even a biweekly check-in call from a friend or workout partner encouraged people to exercise more. It's great to find a friend who will go to the gym with you or hike a mountain on a moment's notice. Fitness friends can challenge you, provide support, offer teamwork, and bring out the competitive side of you. It is important that you find a fitness buddy who will encourage you to be active. A workout pal that is slightly more active than you is even better. This will encourage you to step up your game. Don't pick your best bud who will almost always say, *"Let's skip the gym and grab a drink and breadsticks at Olive Garden."* You need someone who is reliable, positive, slightly competitive, eager, willing to try new things, supportive, and focused on the end goal. If you do not have a fitness buddy yet, do not fret. There are many social avenues where you can find one. Here are some apps and sites to get you started:

Runtastic: This includes live tracking and a cyber-cheering section.

Fitocracy: You can set up a profile, a feed, friending abilities, and updates. You can score points by tracking your workouts and earn badges for certain milestones.

PumpUp: A photo-based social network where you can post goals and share selfies after tough workouts along with other health-related activities.

Strava: An app geared toward cyclists and runners. You can compete with other members and get ranked on a leaderboard.

Fitness Faceoff: You can challenge your friends near and far to be more active than you are.

CHAPTER 14

SUMMARY

- Laugh: it burns calories!

- Look at running a race as an adventure. Soak up the atmosphere, and have fun with it.

- Find a fitness buddy that is trying to accomplish the same goals. Sometimes it can be more fun to exercise with a friend.

CHAPTER 15

Fool Around

"We don't stop playing because we grow old;
we grow old because we stop playing."
—*George Bernard Shaw*

While sitting at a red light, I glance over to my left. On the side of the road, right in out front of the shopping plaza, is a young girl, probably around five years old, waiting for her school bus. She is skipping around the street lamp posts, swinging herself from one post to another. This girl then starts a continuous line of cartwheels down the sidewalk, one after another after without stopping. Her book bag is on both shoulders, and she doesn't seem to care to take it off. She starts with skipping again and heads back towards me. I just admire the big smile on her face. What a life! I glance to the bench what appeared to be this child's mother sitting there. She is watching her daughter but has no prominent smile on her face. Her arms were folded across her chest, as if she was annoyed by what this child is doing. As the light turned green in front of me, I continued on my way just thinking about that scene at the bus stop. We should all go back to being kids. That young girl was having fun! The best part was that she was exercising and didn't act like she hated every second of it. She truly enjoyed what she was doing. Sometimes we have to take the "work" out of workout and instead play, dance, sing, move, and most of all…smile.

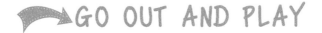

GO OUT AND PLAY

I can remember the phrase used by so many of my teachers: *"Quit monkeying around."* They couldn't wait until recess, and neither could I. And yes, playing around on the monkey bars was the best part of my day! My classmates and I played and didn't think of it as burning calories getting in our thirty minutes of moderate-to-vigorous exercise a day. We were working our growing muscles and didn't even know it. I think of kids running everywhere and parents yelling, *"Slow down," "Stop running,"* and *"Just sit for one minute."* If only we tried to run everywhere like children do. Can you imagine adults darting around the grocery stores just because they loved to zoom from aisle to aisle? It might be a little chaotic, but we would be burning some serious calories and entering hours of activity into our fitness trackers!

If you think back to when you were a child (we were all there at one point), and envision what you would be doing at the park if given the chance, take five minutes and go do it. Some of my best dates with my husband were when we were doing something active like playing hockey on the pond, indoor rock climbing, or zip lining through the trees of the Adirondack Extreme adventure course. The world is our playground. If you have children, let them be part of your fitness. Lead by example. Run and chase them around, push them on the swings, go on the seesaw, skip with them at the bus stop. Don't be the mom or dad that sits there on the park bench texting all day while their kids are playing (not that you need kids to go play at the park, I might add). Be authentic and natural. As Dr. Stuart Brown says in his national bestseller *Play: How It Shapes the Brain, Opens the Imagination, and Invigorates the Soul*: *"Authentic play comes from deep down inside us. It's not formed or motivated solely by others. Real play interacts with and involves the outside world, but it fundamentally expresses the needs and desires of the player. It emerges from the imaginative force within. That's part of the adaptive power of play: with a pinch of pleasure, it integrates deep physiological, emotional, and cognitive capacities"* (104). So seriously…let go and go play. Here are a few fun ideas:

□ Go for a bike ride.
□ Take a hike.
□ Wrestle with your dog!
□ Jump rope.
□ Run up bleachers or stadium stairs.
□ Hula hoop.

☐ Try the monkey bars again.

☐ Go on the swings (great core workout).

☐ Do some leg extensions or tricep dips on the benches.

☐ Climb a tree.

☐ Go roller skating or rollerblading.

☐ Play a game of tennis.

☐ Fly a kite.

☐ Hop on the trampoline.

☐ Geocache- similar to a good old-fashioned treasure hunt!

Whatever you decide, just get out there and play like a kid.

GIVE GAMING A TRY

Video games can be a good thing, if used to stay active! Sitting in front of the television all day may not be a smart choice, but sweating in front of your television, now that's a different story. Check out some of the cool games out there geared to get you moving in front of the screen.

>> Xbox 360: The Xbox 360 has a game called *Your Shape: Fitness Evolved*. This game will offer you kick-butt workouts, fitness plans, and performance trackers to make sure you have good form during your exercises. The game measures your body size and structure, and you can also enter your age, weight, and exercise habits

so it can challenge, but not overexert you. There is an on-screen instructor who leads you through the movements and gives you a score for your performance.

≫ Other game options for the Xbox 360 are *EA Sports Active 2,* which includes a heart rate monitor and nine-week exercise program; *The Biggest Loser Ultimate Workout* with Jillian Michaels and Bob Harper; and *Kinect Sports,* which includes bowling, table tennis, volleyball, track & field, boxing and football. It is fun for the whole family and will not allow you to sit on the couch. You have to get up and move.

≫ WiiFit Plus: This is a great Nintendo workout. This game uses a scale-like controller and balance board. You can customize your fitness, get weighed, and even calculate your body mass index. The game includes over forty types of training (yoga, weight-lifting, balance, and mini-games) for all fitness levels.

≫ Goji Play: When you purchase this wireless sensor, you can use your device to make your workout fun. There are tons of free games and apps to choose from. Your screen will show your real-time fitness metrics during your exercise. Personalize your account, and set goals.

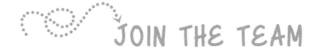

JOIN THE TEAM

MaryAnne and Ed recently purchased a house in The Villages, Florida. They decided that the winters in the Northeast were getting old (and cold!) and that they'd rather enjoy the sunshine during those winter months, instead of sitting around wishing they could ride the golf cart. While wintering in Florida, they discovered a new love—a game called pickle ball. I had never heard of pickle ball before I visited them in Florida. Pickle ball is a sport that uses a court and combines aspects of ping pong, badminton, and tennis. It is played with a paddle and a plastic ball. It is a game for all ages and all levels depending on the team you join. They started by playing a few games with their friends, but soon it turned into a regular thing and became their exercise of choice. Who knew? They have met great friends by playing pickup games and continue to perfect their skill. Now that they are back in town for the summer, they have searched for and successfully found pickle ball courts near their house.

The point I am trying to make is that team "sit-on-the-couch-and-veg-out" is old news. It's time to join a new, active team with the *"Put me in coach, I'm ready to play"* attitude. For those of you wanting to find your inner athlete, discover your competitive side, meet new people, stay active, and have fun at the same time, this avenue may be a great option for you. It does not have to be a whole new sport (though it is fun to explore new things). Perhaps you were a basketball player during your school days and miss the sport. If you still desire to play, find others that love and miss the game, too. Those people are out there—you may just not know how to find them. A little research on the leagues and sports teams in your area will go a long way.

□ Take a trip to your local YMCA. They usually have a list of the recreation leagues and activities in the area.
□ For teams in your area, check out sites like www.playtennis.com, www.kickball.com, and www.softballleagues.net
□ Visit www.sportsvite.com to find partners and players or organize games and teams.
□ Check out bulletin boards at your gym. Rec teams sometimes post when they are looking for teammates.

CHAPTER 15

SUMMARY

- Introduce an element of play into your exercise routine. Be a kid at heart, and enjoy what you are doing.

- Use video games in an active way. You can still be "a gamer" without sitting your butt on the couch!

- Try participating in a team sport instead of watching one on TV. It's never too late to learn a new sport or relive your glory days.

CHAPTER 16

Go Dancing

"Dancers are the athletes of God."
—Albert Einstein

Dancing with your partner can not only be sexy, it can be fun too. Couch could never dance with me, and it was one thing I hated about him. If you feel like you are lacking the motivation, and it takes everything in your power to peel yourself away from Couch, consider this: A recent study in *Social Psychological and Personality Science* revealed that people felt more powerful after listening to a song with heavy bass as opposed to fast tracks. They say that these tunes give people a sense of strength during a challenging task. Isn't it exciting you can get yourself pumped up for exercise with no DJ required? Haven't you ever wondered what happens to your body as soon as you slip those headphones on?

I have witnessed the power of music with my own exercise and continue to watch my clients experience this as well. I have playlists for all of my clients, and I always ask them about their favorite songs and genres. One client in particular is very motivated by music. When she appears to be unable to do any more repetitions, and her form begins to slip, something weird happens: the song changes and she musters up the power to do a few more repetitions. She sings and dances, happy as can be. Her mood changes from fatigue and ready to quit to *"Let's keep going, I got this!"* I know that with her, all I need is a great playlist, and she will rock the workout with flying colors, and push herself to the max. Music inspires and, when used during your workout, will provide so many benefits and encourage you to push through.

STEP TO THE BEAT

The tempo, also known as the beats per minute (bpm) of our workout tunes, is more of a motivator than we are even aware of. The music you choose for your exercise playlist depends on how fast or slow you move. Here is a basic guide to start with:

>> **Bpm <100:** Best suited for slow, relaxation exercises such as yoga, Pilates, or stretching. Examples: "All I Want is You" by U2 *or* "Unwritten" by Natasha Bedingfield.

>> Bpm 120-140: Best suited for a moderate intensity exercise like a brisk walk, jog, or bike ride. Examples: "I Got A Feeling" by Black Eyed Peas or "Beat It" by Michael Jackson.

>> Bpm 130-160: Best suited for high intensity workouts such as plyometric training, some dancing, martial arts, and weight lifting. Examples: "Spiderwebs" by No Doubt or "Hey Ya" by OutKast.

>> Bpm > 160: Intense training or fast running training programs. Examples: "Runnin' Down A Dream" by Tom Petty or "Here I Go Again On My Own" by White Snake.

One thing I have my clients do when they are getting started is download or pick five songs that get them motivated for activity. This is the playlist they use when I am not with them. I tell them to move for the entire length of their playlist. The rules are that the playlist has to be at least ten minutes and you have to exercise during the entire thing. It's an amazing tool because my clients will start out with the mentality that they only have to exercise to the playlist (which they enjoy), but they end up doing more. The music gets them going, and the feeling of accomplishing the task keeps them going. I challenge you to start with three songs or five minutes. Grab your headphones, and get those tunes rocking!

Some apps and tools that can help you get started are:

Pandora: Create an account and enter a bpm depending on your activity. They have power workout, yoga channels, and everything in-between. Find one that motivates you and get your groove on.

PaceDj: This app helps you find the best workout and running songs that will play on your device.

HAVE A DANCE PARTY

Remember dancing along with your friends when your favorite song came on the radio? It may have started off with Journey's "Don't Stop Believing" and turned into an 80's dance party for the next hour and a half. I've had workouts like this, starting with basic step aerobics and ending in a full-out dance party in my client's living room. Another event I often witness is epic dance moves along with torched calories at wedding receptions. People get up and dance for hours. It doesn't matter if they have bad knees or herniated discs. They twist and shout with the best of them! The shoes come off and the sweat starts pouring. No one thinks of this as exercise. They think of this as a good time. Try coming home from a tough day at work and throwing one of your favorite upbeat songs on. It's hard to be in a bad mood when you have a familiar, favorite tune cranking. Amazing how it never gets old!

Dancing can preserve your brainpower, improve your outlook, grow your social circle, and protect your organs. You are hardwired to sync your movements to music, says Costos Karageorghis, PhD, a music and sports researcher and co-author of *Inside Sport Psychology*. Costos notes that moving to the beat is an instinctive response. A study in *Circulation: Heart Failure* found that people with cardiac conditions who danced for just 20 minutes, three times a week saw their heart health improve significantly more than those who stuck with traditional cardio workouts. Dancing can also preserve motor skills, lower the risk of dementia, decrease depression, and help keep your skeleton strong (according to the *National Osteoporosis Foundation*). Try cutting a rug while cleaning your house or hit the nightclubs. Use your living room for your new love: dancing, a.k.a….exercise!

TAKE A CLASS

Whether you have a passion for dance or have no idea how to step to a beat, there are dance classes out there for all levels. That's the beauty of it. I have listed a few of the newer raves below to inspire you to get your groove on. There are more dance classes than you could imagine, so start here and pick one to try based on your specific needs.

>> Zumba: This is best if you want to burn serious calories and throw a little hip action and sexy salsa in there.

>> **Nightclubs:** This is the best DIY workout for a night out on the town and a great way to relieve stress. No organization, just fun.

>> **Pole Dancing:** This is best if you want to build total body strength and work on your gymnastics. A little embarrassment and laughter makes for a fun night out with your best pals.

>> **Ballroom Dancing or Swing:** This is a great class for bonding with your significant other or if you need an idea for date nights.

>> **Line dancing:** This is best for beginners. The beat is repetitive and the moves are typically easy to follow.

>> **Dance, Dance Revolution:** This is best if you want to dance in the comfort of your own home; it also satisfies the inner gamer.

>> **Barre:** This is best for the ballet enthusiast or those who would like to work on flow, flexibility, and smaller stabilizing muscles.

>> **AirBarre:** This is for the aerial gymnast at heart. Go defy gravity!

» **Belly Dancing:** This is a great dance option for those looking to tone hips, pelvis, and deep core muscles while using low impact moves. It is less straining on the joints.

» **Bollywood:** This is best if you are looking for foot-stomping, fast-paced dance moves. It combines some folk and hip-hop moves to Hindi pop beats.

» **Bhangra:** If you are looking for a low-impact cardio workout, this class is for you. This uses traditional folk dance from Northern India.

CHAPTER 16

SUMMARY

- Find music that will motivate you to exercise. Use the appropriate beats per minute based on your exercise modality.

- Dance in your kitchen. That's it! A pretty simple but fun, awesome exercise (not to mention, a stress reliever).

- Find a dance class that seems perfect for you and sign up. It never hurts to try.

CHAPTER 17

Relax

"Tension is who you think you should be.
Relaxation is who you are."
—*Chinese Proverb*

You may be thinking, *"What in the world does relaxing have to do with exercising?"* I know it seems weird, but relaxing can make or break your commitment to moving more. You may also be surprised to know that relaxing does not have to involve Couch either! You see, the purpose of this final part of the book is to show you exercise can be FUN! Sometimes we take ourselves too seriously and need to learn to RELAX for a change. Relaxing can mean taking a day off of training to let your muscles build strength. Relaxing can also mean sinking further into your yoga pose or stretch. Listen to the instructor telling you, *"reeeelaaaax."* Relaxing should not only envelop the physical sense, but also the mental sense. Mental relaxation can lead to more desire for physical activity as well. Zoning out with Couch in front of the TV at the end of a stressful day (which, let's be honest, can be every day if your work gives you stress) will actually do more harm than good. It's better to activate the body's natural relaxation response. Techniques such as deep breathing exercises and meditation can boost your mood and find energy just when you thought you had none left.

SAVOR THE MOMENT

The act of mindfulness is that of enabling yourself to be totally aware and present. The term *"meditation"* can scare people, mostly because it is misunderstood. When I first heard of meditation, I thought it was only used in yoga or by those who practiced Buddhism. Meditation and being mindful offer an ongoing list of physiological, emotional, and spiritual benefits. Visit www.ineedmotivation.com for a list of 100 benefits of meditation. What I discovered during my experimentation with meditation was that it involves deliberate concentration and self-awareness. It can take place during prayer, worship, or when you're alone with your own thoughts.

During my first few times meditating, I started my day as I always did—reading my devotional and reflecting on God's word for a few minutes. I finished with a prayer, and headed out the door to start my busy day. Just before I settled down for the evening, I sat on the floor (not on Couch), closed my eyes, and committed to five minutes of "just me." It forced me to calm down and focus on just being. I ended my night with a prayer and my bedtime tea. Big sigh…I believe there is no right or wrong way to meditate. It just depends on how you get yourself to that state of total awareness and relaxation.

Another exercise to help you relax is to breathe deep. Deep-breathing exercises encourage you to relax and bring oxygen around the body and especially to the muscles that need it most. There are many blogs, podcasts, books, apps, magazines, internet sites, YouTube videos, etc. that will give good tips for meditation and deep-breathing exercises for "newbies." There is an app called **Headspace** for beginner meditators; it walks you through some short, guided meditations, and eventually, you can work your way up to longer sessions. There is also Pandora radio which has meditation channels and apps like **Relax Melodies** that play calming music and nature sounds. The best advice I can give here is the same I give with exercise: start small. Find what works for you, what makes you feel good, and do it consistently to see results.

BE AU NATURAL

Look around you. There are no couches found in nature. Studies have found that "green" or outdoor exercise produces significant improvement in mood and self-esteem. The color green is known to rejuvenate us when we are exhausted emotionally, physically, or mentally. It is also considered the color of balance and harmony. Numerous studies suggest being surrounded by greenery is best for boosting your health and performance. It's clear to see why people get depressed during the fall and winter months when everything seems to lose its green color. If it were up to me, I would put plants all around inside of gyms. The plants would increase the air quality and oxygen levels when we need it the most. The scenery of surrounding nature would also help bring the benefits of the outdoors to the inside.

If you are unable to get outdoors for your activity, here are some ways to bring the outdoors to you.

- ☐ Place plants around the space you usually exercise in. The natural surrounding will help you feel at peace.

- ☐ Diffuse scents that bring you energy like lemon and citrus or scents that calm you down like lavender and rosemary. I use Young Living Essential Oils in my diffuser, depending on what I am trying to accomplish that day. These oils are pure and derived from natural sources.

- ☐ Download music and natural sounds for your cool down and flexibility portion. It can help you stretch for longer periods of time and really relax into your stretch.

- ☐ Eat a clean, plant-based diet with organic fruits and vegetables. You can even grow your own spices and vegetables indoors.

☐ **When you can, exercise in your bare feet. It will feel great to be energized, calm, motivated and inspired, all at the same time.**

GIVE THANKS

Having an "attitude of gratitude" does wonders for stress relief. It's good to give thanks all throughout the year and not just on the Thanksgiving holiday. Being grateful builds awareness and reminds us all that we are blessed, no matter what it looks like to the outside world. Thankfulness sparks feelings of positivity and well-being. Think of someone who said *"Thank you"* to you or when you received a hand-written thank-you card in the mail. How did it make you feel? It feels great, right? Giving thanks is such a simple yet powerful way to create positive energy. Psychologists Robert Emmons and Michael McCullough point out that the benefits of expressing gratitude range from better physical health to improved mental alertness. Expressing gratitude may even protect you from certain forms of psychological disorders. Practice saying THANK YOU to others, even if it's for a small thing. Perhaps they hold the door for you, pass along their shopping cart, or let you merge into their traffic lane. Be grateful for these moments, and be sure to say thanks.

A few ways you can practice being more grateful is to find small things to be thankful for and write them down.

Include material things, abilities, people, and situations you are grateful for, and be sure to expand on why. For example: I am grateful for my house. It is warm and cozy, and I love the memories we are building in it. Get the family involved. Read it at the dinner table, or share it over a cup of coffee. Last year our family put *"I am thankful for_____"* notes in our stockings and read them all on Christmas day. It was amazing, and we continue to do this throughout the year. It opens the heart and brings positive vibes to the people we care about. Go be thankful for your healthy body and the freedom to exercise when you chose to do so. You can use websites and apps mentioned in *USA Today* and on NPR like **Gratitude Journal** and **Gratitude Journal 365** to help you rewire your brain and get you to a place of happiness and gratefulness.

SLEEP WITH ME

Nighty Night. Sleep tight. Dream of healthy changes tonight. Sleep is an important part of any relationship. Just ask my husband and kids. If I don't get my peaceful sleep, I am not the best person I could possibly be in the morning! According to a recent Gallup Poll, 40% of Americans get just six hours of sleep each night. No wonder we have to deal with Ms. Cranky Pants in the office every morning. Lack of sleep causes a slew of health problems. The issues I would like to mention are weight gain, moodiness, and an overall sluggishness. If you are exhausted, it may make it harder for you to exercise or resist temptations when they come along. Sleep heals the body and hits your reset button. If you cut your hours short, you may not be able to completely refresh the system.

According to the National Sleep Foundation, there are sleep recommendations for every age group. Visit sleepfoundation.org for the full chart of recommendations. For the purpose of this book, I will leave newborns up to the age of 13 out of the conversation. Here are the recommended hours of uninterrupted sleep you should be getting in a 24 hour period:

Ages 14-17: 8-10 hours of sleep
Ages 18-25: 7-9 hours of sleep
Ages 26-64: 7-9 hours of sleep
Ages 65+:   7-8 hours of sleep

Does this surprise you? Of course everyone is different so you may feel that you need more or less depending on your own individual needs. If you feel that you are not getting enough sleep, you may want to give the following simple ideas a try.

☐ Turn off and silence all devices and electronics an hour or two before bedtime.
☐ Dim the lights in your bedroom before bed.
☐ Take a hot bath or shower.
☐ Practice deep breathing.
☐ Listen to calming music.

☐ Diffuse calming essential oils that promote relaxation (lavender and Roman chamomile).

☐ Use your bed for sleep and sex. Oh, and have sex! This releases endorphins (those "feel good" hormones) and creates a sense of calm afterwards, due to the lack of the stress hormone, cortisol.

☐ Go to bed five minutes earlier than you usually do. This will add up to thirty five extra minutes of sleep each week. Every bit counts!

☐ If you like background noise while you sleep, try apps like Bed Time Fan or White Noise Ambience Lite.

☐ Is it time for a new mattress or pillow? Aches and pains when you wake up and endless nights of tossing and turning means you may want to reevaluate what you are sleeping on. You can get as expensive as you want here. There are mattresses and pillows that track your sleep and even give you massages! It may just be time to invest in some new zzzzzzs.

GO WITH THE FLOW

Water, as we all know, is a vital part of life. Our bodies are made of 90% water. Our muscles are made up of 70-75% water. It makes sense that water can energize our muscles when we have enough of it; likewise, we can understand why we can't perform at our peak when we have inadequate fluids stored up in our powerhouse. Water is a miracle cure for a slew of ailments—not to mention all its other great benefits. What does this have to do with having fun? Well, if you are sluggish, moody, and not motivated, that does not sound like fun at all! Not drinking enough water might be your issue. Easy enough to fix, right?

People often ask the question, *"How much water should I be drinking daily?"* The simple answer is to take your weight and divide it in half. That is the number of ounces you should be consuming just for normal daily function. For example, I weigh 140 pounds so I need to consume 70 ounces of water daily. Naturally, you will need more than that if you are exercising and exerting yourself. Replacing fluids lost during perspiration is equally as important as drinking enough in the first place. A great app to log your water intake is **Water Time Pro**. It sends you cute little reminders throughout the day to keep you on track. You could also start a hydration calendar or use your food diary to keep track of your intake. Drink up, and notice how great you start to feel. Add some fresh fruit or carbonation to change it up.

Water is also an advantageous exercise environment itself. It's wonderful for taking the stress off of your joints. That is why aquatic exercise is one of the best choices for the injured, elderly, overweight, athletes-in-training, and pretty much everyone. Try not to smile while you are floating around on a noodle, doing a cannonball, or tossing around a beach ball. I am willing to bet you can't. Water is not only FUN to play in, it is FUN-ctional as well. What a way to jumpstart your fitness!

Lastly, water is soothing to listen to. Sound machines and spas play sounds of the ocean and running water to encourage a deeper relaxation. I feel like it is a sound that soothes the soul. Take advantage of Mother Nature and embrace her most valuable resource: it may be your golden ticket to a healthier, more vivacious life.

TRUST YOURSELF

Once upon a time, there were a bunch of tiny frogs who arranged a running competition. The goal was to reach the top of a very high tower. A big crowd gathered around the tower to see the race and cheer on the contestants. No one in crowd believed that the tiny frogs would reach the top of the tower. Statements like, *"Oh, Waaaaay too difficult!"* or *"They will never make it to the top!"* or *"Not a chance that they will succeed"* could be heard (even, *"The tower is too high!"*). The tiny frogs began collapsing one by one, except for those, who in a fresh tempo, climbed higher and higher. The crowd continued to yell, *"It is too difficult! No one will make it!"*

More tiny frogs became tired and gave up but one frog continued higher and higher and higher. This one just wouldn't give up. At the end, everyone else had given up climbing the tower except for the one tiny frog who, after a big effort, was the only one who reached the top. Then all of the other tiny frogs naturally wanted to know how this one frog managed to do it. A contestant asked the winner how he had found the strength to succeed and reach the goal. He couldn't answer the inquisitive contestant because it turned out that the frog who had won was deaf.

The parable of the frog conveys the message that if you believe in yourself, you will achieve great things. Your body achieves what the mind believes. You will become what you believe if your belief is strong enough. Countless examples of this are seen throughout history, dating back to Jesus Christ himself. The concept is not new—it just needs to be emphasized here. Like anything else in life, yes, there will be struggles; yes, there will be obstacles. Said best out of the mouth of Henry Ford, *"Whether you think you can or you think you can't, you're right."* Create your belief statement. Take a mental picture and frame it. Believe and prove that you absolutely CAN and WILL say goodbye to the dominating Couch in your life for good.

CHAPTER 17

SUMMARY

✓ Take time out of your day to practice being mindful. Meditate and build awareness of your healthy body and mind.

✓ Go green. Exercise as much as you can outdoors, and when you are unable, bring the outdoors in to you.

✓ Be sure to give daily thanks for your many blessings. Focus on what you have and not on what you don't have.

✓ Use methods for getting a better quality night's sleep. This will allow you to be more energized and ready for what the day has to offer.

✓ Use the powers of water to energize, motivate, stimulate, and relax your body.

✓ Believe that you can do anything you put your mind to, and you will achieve great things.

A Fairytale Ending

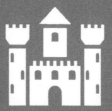

Dear Reader,

Couch is now officially your ex. It was hard at first, but you powered through it and did what was best for you. I am glad to know that you and Couch are good friends but have no desire to date each other ever again. I hear that you and your new love, Exercise, are due to be married and will soon say those special words, "until death do us part." You have the best years of your life ahead of you. Congratulations on your happily ever after!

Keep it simple,
    explore what's possible,
        & trust the journey

Jenn

CONCLUSION

A Fairytale Ending

We live in a microwave society-we want quick fixes and we want them now! It's hard to look at the end goal and imagine the time and amount of work it will take to get there. That's enough to get people to not even start. Small, consistent changes trump all things. If you understand that it will take some time to build a healthy lifestyle and that you must be willing to try, then you are more than halfway there. Find one healthy change you can incorporate into your life starting today. Start small, move more, and you will see results. They may not be visible at first, but internally, things are changing. Change is not an event, it's a process. As Tony Robbins writes in *Unlimited Power*: *"Those who succeed are committed to changing and being flexible until they do create the life that they desire"* (13). Be bold, step out, and never quit.

The purpose of this book is to provide ideas of things to try, tools to use, and perhaps inspiration to get you moving. I understand that we all have different goals, motivations, and ideas that inspire—we are all vastly unique packages. Sometimes we try something, it doesn't work, and we must move on. Thomas Edison put it best: *"I have not failed, I've simply discovered ten thousand ways that don't work."* Failure means that you are trying. Failure means that you are taking risks and putting yourself out there. If the suggestions I have provided in this book have not worked for you, find others. Don't stop here.

There is always a way; it's never too late to start fresh and do things differently. Take some time to explore what it is you really want in life. Take time to focus on your dreams and talk to people about how to achieve them. Find people that can help you. It's amazing the people that want to be there for you. We are all on this earth for our God-given purpose. You are meant to truly live and enjoy your time here. This is your time to reinvent yourself. Conquering exercise will make you feel like you can do anything in all aspects of life. You will feel better and be a happier, healthier person because of it. I encourage you to get up and get moving. Don't sit around and let life pass you by. This is your journey, and there is no better time to start than right now. Write your own story, and be prepared for your fairytale ending. If you don't know where to start, try *My Healthy Life Journal* available on Amazon. It will help you build the habit of small, simple changes each and every day.

Visit jennbenson.com for more resources,
downloadable content, and worksheets that go
along with this book. You can also download
*The Ultimate Resource Guide To Breaking Up
with Your Couch* found on the homepage of
jennbenson.com website.
Be sure to join the the couch busting tribe and
receive weekly emails with fun challenges to
help you leave couch for good!

If you found this book helpful and want to share
all about it, please leave a review on the web
from wherever you purchased the book.

Recommended

Readings

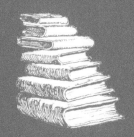

RECOMMENDED

Readings

"In a good book, the best is between the lines."
—*Swedish Proverb*

Bakker, Frank C., Boschker, Marc S.J.,& Chung, Tjuling. (1996). Changes In Muscular Activity While Imagining Weight Lifting Using Similar Response Propositions. *Journal of Sport & Exercise Psychology,* Vol. 18, 313-24.

Batmanghelidj, F. *Your Body's Many Cries for Water.* Global Health Solutions, Inc., 2008.

Baumeister, Roy F. and John Tierney. *Willpower: Rediscovering the Greatest Human Strength.* Penguin Books, 2011.

Brue, Suzanne. *the 8 colors of fitness: Use the power of self-understanding to live a more physically active life.* Delray Beach, Oakledge Press, 2008.

Brown, Stuart & Vaughan, Christopher. *Play: How It Shapes the Brain, Opens the Imagination, and Invigorates the Soul.* Penguin, 2009.

Cialdini, Robert. *Influence: The Psychology of Persuasion.* Harper Collins, 2007.

Cooper, Robert K. *Get Out Of Your Own Way.* Advanced Excellence Systems, 2006.

Covey, Stephen R. *The 7 Habits of Highly Effective People: Powerful Lessons in Personal Change.* FreePress, 2004.

Duhigg, Charles. *The Power Of Habit: Why We Do What We Do In Life And Business.* Random House, 2014.

Dyer, Wayne W. *Excuses Begone!: How to Change Lifelong, Self-Defeating Thinking Habits.* Hay House, Inc., 2009.

Emmons, Robert A.,& McCullough, Michael E. (February 2003). Counting Blessings Versus Burdens: An Experimental Investigation of Gratitude and Subjective Well-being in Daily Life. *Journal of Personality and Social Psychology*, Vol. 84, No. 2, pp.377-89.

Hill, Napoleon. *Think & Grow Rich.* Barnes and Noble, 2008.

Johnson, Spencer. *Who Moved My Cheese?: An A-Mazing Way to Deal with Change in Your Work and in Your Life.* G.P Putnam's Sons,1998 (p.74).

Kennedy, Robert. *Bull'$ Eye: Targeting Your Life for Real Financial Wealth and Personal Fulfillment.* Robert Kennedy Publishing, 2012.

LaRoche, Loretta. *Life is Short—Wear Your Party Pants: Ten Simple Truths That Lead To An Amazing Life.* Hay House, Inc., 2003.

Levine, James A. *Get Up!: Why Your Chair Is Killing You And What You Can Do About It.* St. Martin's Griffin, 2014.

Nicklaus, Jack. *Golf My Way.* Simon and Schuster Paperbacks, 1974 (p.79).

Peeke, Pamela. *Fit to Live.* Rodale Books, 2007.

Pink, Daniel H. Drive*: The Surprising Truth About What Motivates Us.* Riverhead Books, 2009.

Reynolds, Gretchen. *The First 20 Minutes: Surprising Science Reveals How We Can Exercise Better, Train Smarter, Live Longer.* Hudson Street Press, 2012.

Robbins, Tony. *Unlimited Power: The New Science Of Personal Achievement.* Simon and Schuster, 1986.

Sincero, Jen. *You are Badass: How to Stop Doubting Your Greatness and Start Living an Awesome Life.* Running Press, 2013.

Tracy, Brian. *Goals!: How to Get Everything You Want-Faster Than You Ever Thought Possible.* Berrett-Koehler Publisher Inc., 2010.

Ziglar, Zig. *Better Than Good: Creating a Life You Can't Wait to Live.* Thomas Nelson, 2006.

Recommended
Websites

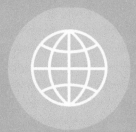

RECOMMENDED WEBSITES

Part One

Getting Started

www.Everydayaffirmations.org
www.Ideafit.com
www.Niketrainingclub.com
www.Psychologytoday.com
www.Self.com
www.Sparkpeople.com
www.Wello.com

RECOMMENDED WEBSITES

Part Two

Staying Motivated

www.Exercisefriends.com

www.Fitnessmeetup.com

www.Goal-setting-for-success.com

www.Hammockwayoflife.com

www.Meetup.com

www.Sensoriafitness.com

www.The8colorsoffitness.com

www.Wikihow.com/Use-the-Footprint-Test.com

RECOMMENDED WEBSITES

Part Three

Having Fun

www.9gag.com

www.Bloodsweatandcheers.com

www.Collegehumor.com

www.Laughteryoga.org

www.Gigglers.tv

www.ineedmotivation.com

www.Kickball.com

www.Playtennis.com

www.Sportsvite.com

www.Strava.com

Recommended

Apps

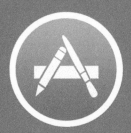

RECOMMENDED APPS

Part One

Getting Started

21 Habit
5 Minute Home Workouts
Awesome Note 2
Beeminder
GymPact (Pact)
Happify
HealthyWage
Map My Run
Move
My Fitness Pal
NexTrack
Nike + Training Club
Pedometer ++
Pocket Life Calendar
Rise
Stand up!

stickK

Talkspace

Thumbtack

Unique Daily Affirmations

Wello

RECOMMENDED APPS

Part Two

Staying Motivated

iBird Pro
iWish
Happy Scale
Happy Tapper
Leafsnap
Lifetick
RootsRated

RECOMMENDED APPS
_____

Part Three
_____

Having Fun

Bed Time Fan
Charity Miles
Fitness Faceoff
Fitocracy
Gratitude Journal
Gratitude Journal 365
Headspace
Missile Wars
PaceDj
Pandora
PumpUp
Relax Melodies
Runtastic
Strava Running and Cycling
Water Time Pro
White Noise Ambience Lite
Zombies, Run!

JENN BENSON

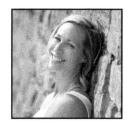

Jenn is a fit inspirationalist, trainer, and health & wellness strategist. Drawing on her training, expertise, and her own personal experience, **Jenn Benson** will help you ease into exercise in a non-intimidating atmosphere. **Jenn's** approach is simple and her easy-to-follow action plan has helped countless people discover their passion for exercise. You can visit her at **www.jennbenson.com**.